Strange Symptom

How I became my own health detective (although I didn't mean to) and how it changed my life completely.

Iryna Khmara

This message is for those of you experiencing strange symptoms, feeling unwell, dealing with multiple diagnoses, and searching for solutions that seem elusive — there is hope. I know because I've been there.

Perhaps this book will assist you on your journey, offering a fresh perspective. You might find your own health story reflected within its pages, along with the support and understanding you've been seeking.

I received this message from kind strangers and from the world around me. Now, I'm sharing it with all of you.

You are not alone.

Disclaimer

Just a friendly reminder: I'm not a doctor, so this book isn't a substitute for professional medical advice. While I've poured my heart into sharing my journey, it's crucial that you consult with your healthcare specialist before diving into blood tests or diagnosing yourself. Your health is unique, and a professional can provide the best guidance tailored to you. Happy reading and stay healthy!

I am filled with immense gratitude for the people who have supported and guided me, who saved my sanity and my life throughout my journey:

Toma

Tony

Masha

Perry

Alyona

Dr. Maliarenko

I will be eternally grateful

With love,

Iryna

I would like to extend my heartfelt thanks to Andrii Tanenkov, my brilliant ebook designer, for his meticulous work in converting this book into its beautiful electronic form. Your expertise and attention to detail have brought this project to life.

Chapter 1

So, my health journey began (yes, by the end I was covered in mud, blood, and sweat, feeling like a hero who had just vanquished a hideous monster) ten years ago when I visited my gynecologist with a concern. Well, it wasn't even a major problem, just a minor issue causing some discomfort in my vagina. As it turned out, it was a vaginal thrush.

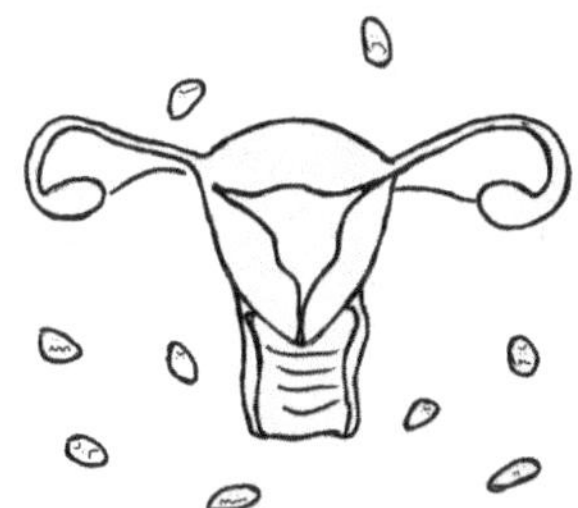

Image 1. Vaginal Thrush

At that time, I was going through a difficult divorce. I had thought that man was the love of my life, but reality proved to be much harsher than I had expected. Then, I fell in love again, and this relationship turned out to be even more ugly. I hadn't healed from my previous traumas and ended up falling into the same pit again.

You see, with absent parents and psychological violence in my childhood, I grew up trying to earn the love that should have been freely given. This pattern led me to a man who was, well, fantastic in the bedroom but an absolute jerk in every other aspect. No mental abuse though, but he was rude enough to be another mistake on my way. Ugh.

So, we broke up — I quit. I started living a quiet life, volunteering, contemplating my next steps, looking for a new job, and healing. I've read lots of psychological stuff, was thinking about going to psychotherapy and learned how to be kind to myself. Then, bam! I met a normal man (someone not from my trauma-riddled past and, therefore, a bit alien to me). I fell in love and thought all my life struggles were finally over.

Well, life has thousands of ways to surprise us. Or overwhelm us. It's all optional, and we can't control everything that comes our way (or can we?).

I was happy, yet simultaneously stressed and anxious. I think my previous experiences added to it, so I got that vaginal thrush, unpleasant thing I have to admit. So, I rushed to see a doctor — a

Vaginal Thrush (Vaginal Candidiasis)

What is Vaginal Thrush?

Vaginal thrush, also known as vaginal candidiasis or yeast infection, is a common fungal infection caused by an overgrowth of Candida, particularly Candida albicans. This yeast is normally present in small amounts in the vagina along with various bacteria, maintaining a healthy balance. However, when this balance is disrupted, Candida can multiply and cause an infection.

Chapter 2

The doctor, a very serious and professional woman who had worked in a state hospital for decades, ran some tests and gave me prescriptions. She also advised me to eat more yogurt in the mornings to add some good bacteria to my body. I hated yogurt before, but I decided to give it a try. I started making homemade yogurt, which turned out to be super healthy and much better than any yogurt from the supermarket or café.

I got better pretty fast and decided to eat dairy products more often. In my family, dairy wasn't really popular. We had some cheese sandwiches from time to time, syrnyky (cottage cheese pancakes — a popular Eastern European food), and my parents used to drink kefir (that disgusting creation of the devil itself that stinks like... like... I don't know what, but I still hate that smell).

My grandmas, on the other hand, were dairy enthusiasts. During our summer visits to the village, we (my sister and I) indulged in various pies, cottage cheese, and fresh milk. Grandpa had cheese and butter every morning, calling his sandwich — a slice of black bread topped with thick butter and cheese — a "marine sandwich." He had this every day during his navy service, where he rose to the rank of captain third class. Naturally, I enjoyed them too.

What is Dairy?

Dairy products come from milk, which is usually from cows but can also come from goats, sheep, and even buffalo. These products are packed with nutrients that help keep our bones strong and our bodies healthy.

Common Dairy Products

1. **Milk:** *The star of the show! Milk can be enjoyed as a refreshing drink or used as a base for many other dairy delights. It's rich in calcium, which is great for your bones and teeth.*

2. **Cheese:** *Cheese comes in so many varieties that it's like a world of its own! From soft and creamy brie to sharp and tangy cheddar, there's a cheese for every taste.*

3. **Yogurt:** *This creamy treat is not only delicious but also good for your tummy. Yogurt is packed with probiotics, which are friendly bacteria that help keep your digestive system happy.*

4. **Butter:** *Made from cream, butter adds a rich and creamy flavor to all kinds of dishes. Whether spread on toast or melted over vegetables, it's a kitchen essential.*

5. **Cream:** *From light cream in your coffee to heavy whipping cream for desserts, this dairy product is all about adding that extra touch of richness to your food.*

Why is Dairy Important?

Dairy products are an excellent source of calcium, vitamin D, and protein. These nutrients are essential for:

- **Strong Bones and Teeth:** *Calcium and vitamin D work together to keep your bones and teeth strong and healthy.*

- **Muscle Growth:** *Protein is the building block of muscles, and dairy products provide a good amount of it.*

- **Energy:** *Dairy products contain various vitamins and minerals that help keep your energy levels up throughout the day.*

Fun Dairy Facts

- **Did you know?** *It takes about 10 pounds of milk to make just 1 pound of cheese!*

- **Fun Fact:** *The most popular cheese in the world is mozzarella, thanks to its starring role on pizza*

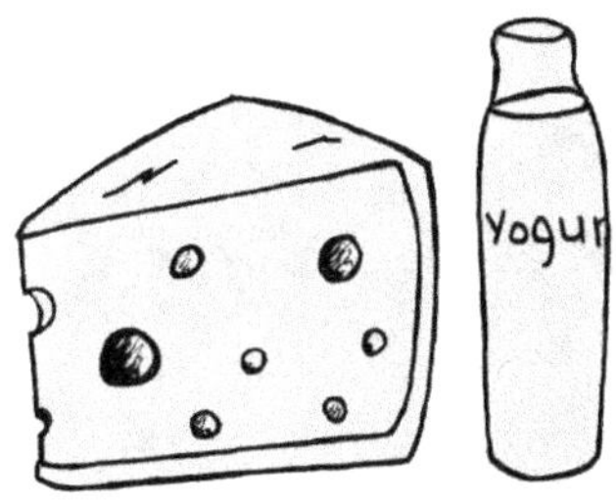

Image 2. Dairy

My new discovery was incredible. Have you ever made a caprese salad with freshly grown basil from your garden? Or a veggie salad with Parmesan? Have you ever tried fresh homemade sugar-free yogurt with berries and fruits? Oh yeah, it was fantastic, and I savored every bite and every day. Yogurt became a significant part of my daily routine, and I was healthy and happy. I forgot about all my problems until The Day I had an emergency surgery.

It was in 2019, and my vaginal thrush was discovered in 2015, I haven't heard from it since, so I had been healthy for four years.

But I don't think I really was.

Chapter 3

The Day and other stories

So, before The Day, I started noticing some weird changes. For instance, every morning after breakfast, my mental state got worse. It was as if I was under immense pressure. It's a very strange sensation when your mind is flooded with thoughts and anxiety, and you can almost "hear" a noise inside your head, like the static of an old TV. This sensation was particularly clear and sharp after having tea or coffee, so I decided to eliminate caffeine from my diet. Some of my friends had this feeling after caffeine, so it was obvious. Or I just thought it was.

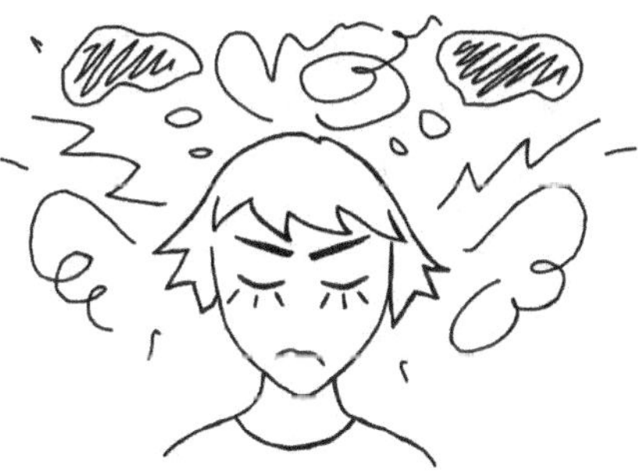

Image 3. Anxiety

My life was amazing at that time. I was making documentaries and meeting fascinating people almost every day, so I wasn't particularly concerned. Initially, this strange sensation was barely noticeable; it crept in gradually, gaining intensity day by day, slowly. In such a situation, you get used to it and don't really notice the incremental changes.

In 2017, during the spring allergy season, I started feeling exceptionally bad. I took my usual antihistamines, which alleviated the symptoms. Typically, my allergies involved nasal issues, occasional coughing, and breathing problems during the tree bloom. The small pills, along with nose drops, usually worked wonders. But if I didn't take them, I could have had bronchitis or worse (as in childhood years).

But in 2017, I felt like I had the flu. My body was heavy, and I experienced fatigue, weakness, and an overall sense of illness. Occasionally, a strange hot wave would course through my body. However, antihistamines worked, and by summer, I had completely forgotten about these issues.

Antihistamines

Antihistamines are a class of medications that counteract the effects of histamine, a chemical released by the immune system during allergic reactions. Histamine binds to receptors on certain cells, causing symptoms like itching, swelling, and vasodilation (widening of blood vessels). Antihistamines block these receptors, thereby alleviating allergy symptoms.

Mechanism of Action

Antihistamines work by blocking histamine receptors, specifically the H1 receptors, on cells in the body. Histamine, when released during an allergic reaction, binds to these receptors and causes symptoms such as itching, sneezing, runny nose, and watery eyes. By preventing histamine from binding to its receptors, antihistamines reduce or eliminate these symptoms.

The same situation occurred in 2018 and 2019. Each spring, I felt progressively worse, beyond the usual allergy symptoms. However, the antihistamines remained effective, allowing me to continue with my daily life. But in 2019, something changed. Alongside the persistent white noise in my head, I experienced chronic fatigue. I felt heavy and constantly tired, since March. Additionally, I began to suffer from severe nausea whenever I traveled, whether in a car or a bus – it didn't matter which vehicle; I felt intensely sick. Then, on May 19th, as far as I remember, the incident happened.

I was stepping out of the bathroom when I felt a sudden, intense pain in my lower abdomen. The pain was excruciating, as if something had just exploded inside me. My limbs turned to jelly, I was trembling, and my skin turned as pale as a sheet of paper (I never thought that phrase was more than a literary cliché, but my reflection in the mirror resembled a zombie). I staggered to the sofa, trying to pull myself together, but I don't know how anyone manages that in such situations. For a moment I became a super-human and could drag myself to that sofa, but I have no idea HOW I did that.

Panic surged through my body, and I was about to call an ambulance, but suddenly — bam! — the pain vanished, and I felt normal again. "O-o-kaaay!" I told myself, and went on to pack my things since I was traveling back home that day. A few hours later, I was on the train, feeling fine, with no trace of nausea. The pain and fear seemed like a distant memory. However, when I got home, had dinner, and went to bed, the pain returned with a vengeance.

But it was deeper and more disturbing; it felt like I was on my period, but the place that period occupies inside you now was EVERYWHERE inside my belly. Ambulance it was, and that night I had emergency surgery.

It was a cyst rupture. No one could explain to me why the cyst appeared there in the first place. The only explanation I got was, "You are a woman, you know, the hormones and such, no one knows why cysts may occur. There could be numerous reasons — hormonal fluctuations, stress, and so forth — so it is what it is. Recover, and everything will be okay. Visit your gynecologist."

What are Ovarian Cysts?

Ovarian cysts are fluid-filled sacs or pockets that develop on or inside an ovary. Most ovarian cysts are harmless and go away on their own without treatment. However, some can cause symptoms and may require medical attention.

Causes of Ovarian Cysts

- **Hormonal Imbalances:** *Issues with the hormonal system that controls ovulation.*

- **Pregnancy:** *Some ovarian cysts form early in pregnancy to support the pregnancy until the placenta forms.*

- **Endometriosis:** *Endometrial tissue can attach to the ovary and form a cyst.*
- **Severe Pelvic Infections:** *Infections can spread to the ovaries and cause cysts.*

So I started my recovery. I was feeling fine physically, but mentally I was a bit shaken. The doctors told me it was normal to feel a bit off after surgery, and I took their word for it. I focused on getting back to my routines, eating healthy, and trying to keep my stress levels low.

Of course, I recovered, but I was really shocked by the situation and decided to visit a gynecologist to check my hormones again. Surprisingly, they were fine. It's the strangest thing that can happen, right? The gynecologist proposed taking birth control pills to prevent any future "hormonal imbalances," but I refused. It just didn't feel right for me, even though I'm not against them in general. She also suggested that I should consider having a baby, her tone and expression clearly indicating it should be as soon as possible.

Birth Control Pills

Birth control pills, also known as oral contraceptives, are medications taken by mouth to prevent pregnancy. They are one of the most popular and effective methods of contraception when used correctly.

Types of Birth Control Pills

There are two main types of birth control pills:

1. **Combination Pills:**

   - **Components:** *Contain both estrogen and progestin hormones.*

   - **Mechanism:** *These hormones work together to prevent ovulation (the release of an egg from the ovaries). They also thicken the mucus in the cervix, making it harder for sperm to reach an egg, and thin the lining of the uterus, making it less likely for a fertilized egg to implant.*

   - **Types:**

     - **Monophasic:** *Each active pill contains the same dose of hormones.*

     - **Multiphasic:** *The hormone levels in the active pills vary, often designed to mimic the natural menstrual cycle.*

2. **Progestin-Only Pills (Mini-Pills):**

   - **Components:** *Contain only progestin.*

   - **Mechanism:** *Primarily work by thickening cervical mucus and thinning the uterine lining. They may also sometimes suppress ovulation.*

   - **Uses:** *Often recommended for women who cannot take estrogen, such as those who are breastfeeding or have certain health conditions.*

Benefits

- **Pregnancy Prevention:** *Highly effective at preventing pregnancy.*

- **Regulated Menstrual Cycles:** *Can make periods more regular and lighter.*

- **Reduced Menstrual Cramps:** *Often decreases the severity of menstrual cramps.*

- **Acne Improvement:** *Can help reduce acne in some women.*

- **Reduced Risk of Certain Cancers:** *Long term use has been associated with a reduced risk of ovarian and endometrial cancers.*

- **Management of Menstrual Disorders:** *Can help manage conditions like endometriosis, polycystic ovary syndrome (PCOS), and premenstrual dysphoric disorder (PMDD).*

Why did I add those details here? To show you that I didn't have polycystic ovary syndrome. My ovary cyst was a one-time, random occurrence with no other cysts present. My cycle had been stable since I was 14, I didn't have endometriosis, I wasn't planning to get pregnant, and I didn't have acne.

I was just tired, anxious, and experienced strange allergy symptoms during spring. Yet, I was proposed to take birth control pills to prevent something doctors couldn't definitively say I had or might have in the future.

At that moment, I realized that doctors (as all the other human beings) can act like they have no idea what they're doing. Just like all of us. It's normal. But if you're searching for help as a patient, you might lose your trust in medicine in such a situation and turn to random remedies like drinking strange herbal concoctions or even becoming religious, swearing off doctor's offices forever (until the next crisis, of course).

But I didn't do that. I'm sure that medicine can make miracles, you just need to find the right doctor.

I was visiting my psychotherapist once a week, trying to get my life back on track. I put that cyst on the "random events" shelf. Moreover, my nausea was gone, and I felt much better. However, the white noise in my head persisted, and anxiety continued to build up.

Chapter 4

I'm from Eastern Europe, and here all women's problems are solved with the baby spell. You're exhausted? Clearly, it's because you don't have a baby. If you had one, you'd never feel tired again (says your friend who hasn't slept for months and is perpetually yelling at her kids). Relationship issues with your husband? Divorce? Unthinkable! You need to have a baby together, and magically, all your problems will vanish! (I'm not kidding, folks, this was the actual advice I received when I planned to divorce my first husband).

Feeling unwell? Plagued by dark thoughts? Suicidal ideations? Oh no, that's concerning! The solution? A baby! A baby will be your savior; you'll be so engrossed with the demands of parenthood that you'll have zero time for yourself, let alone any existential musings!

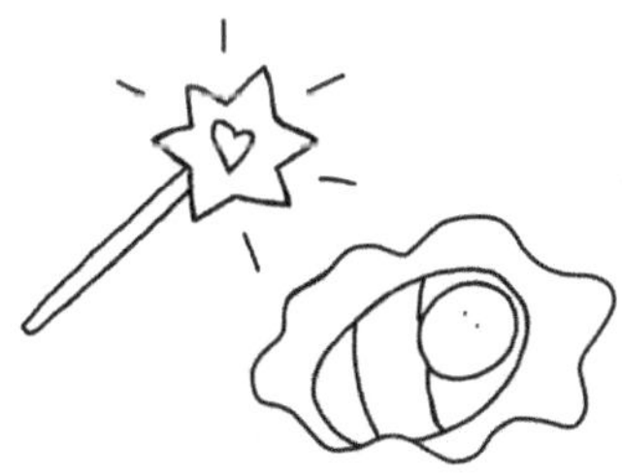

Image 4. The Baby Spell

Your breasts hurt? They're full of cysts?! Oh no! You need a baby! Give birth and all your breast problems will magically vanish! – said the gynecologist, and then another ultrasound specialist, and then another gynecologist. I ran away from the first one like she was a monster. Well, considering her advice, maybe she really was.

But how did I end up in this situation in the first place? Well, it started with my breasts hurting. It was about a year after the surgery, and I noticed this strange, nagging pain. My breasts were swollen and bigger than usual. Sure, it's normal for women to experience this before their period or even mid cycle. But this pain wasn't tied to my cycle at all. It was random. So, I decided to get an ultrasound at the state clinic. The doctor spent 20 minutes examining my breasts and then dropped the bombshell: "You need to visit your gynecologist because you have cysts all over your breasts."

I was terrified. I had no idea such a thing existed, so I ran to my gynecologist. Then I visited another one. You can guess how that went. Not great. They all hit me with the "baby spell" advice.

I googled tons of information about pregnancy, breast issues, and all sorts of related topics. The more I read, the more absurd her advice seemed. It was like she was suggesting I cure a finger pain by stitching a new one to my hand — a metaphor, but you get the drift. Her solution was wildly disproportionate to the problem at hand. I couldn't believe this was the best medical advice available.

Negative Impacts of Giving Birth on a Woman's Health

While childbirth is a natural process, it can have several negative impacts on a woman's health, both in the short term and long term. These effects can vary widely depending on individual circumstances, the mode of delivery, and any pre-existing health conditions.

Physical Impacts

1. ***Vaginal Tears and Episiotomy***

   - ***Vaginal Tears:*** *During vaginal delivery, the perineum (the area between the vagina and anus) can tear. Tears can vary from minor to severe, with severe tears potentially affecting the muscles of the rectum and requiring surgical repair.*

   - ***Episiotomy:*** *Sometimes, a surgical cut (episiotomy) is made in the perineum to facilitate delivery, which can cause pain and take time to heal.*

2. ***Cesarean Section (C-Section) Complications***

   - ***Surgical Risks:*** *As with any surgery, a C-section carries risks such as infection, bleeding, and adverse reactions to anesthesia.*

   - ***Recovery:*** *Recovery from a C-section is generally longer and more painful than recovery from vaginal delivery.*

3. ***Pelvic Floor Dysfunction***

   - ***Incontinence:*** *Damage to the pelvic floor muscles during childbirth can lead to urinary or fecal incontinence.*

   - ***Prolapse:*** *There is also a risk of pelvic organ prolapse, where organs such as the bladder or uterus descend into or outside of the vaginal canal.*

4. **Postpartum Hemorrhage**
   - **Excessive Bleeding:** *Some women experience severe bleeding after childbirth, which can be life-threatening if not managed promptly.*

5. **Infections**
   - **Uterine Infections:** *Infections of the uterus, particularly after a C-section, can occur and may require antibiotics or further medical intervention.*
   - **Mastitis:** *Breastfeeding mothers can develop mastitis, an infection of the breast tissue.*

Emotional and Mental Health Impacts

1. **Postpartum Depression**
   - *Symptoms: Includes severe mood swings, exhaustion, and a sense of hopelessness. This condition can affect the mother's ability to care for her baby and herself.*
   - *Prevalence: Affects about 1 in 9 women according to the CDC.*

2. **Postpartum Anxiety**
   - *Symptoms: Excessive worry, irritability, and restlessness. This can be overwhelming and may interfere with daily functioning.*

3. **Post-Traumatic Stress Disorder (PTSD)**
   - *Causes: Traumatic birth experiences, such as emergency C-sections or significant complications, can lead to PTSD.*

Long-Term Health Impacts

1. ***Chronic Pain***

   - ***Pelvic Pain:*** *Some women experience chronic pelvic pain long after childbirth.*

   - ***Back Pain:*** *Ongoing back pain can result from changes in posture and muscle strain during pregnancy and delivery.*

2. **Hormonal Changes**

   - **Thyroid Issues:** *Pregnancy can affect thyroid function, leading to conditions like postpartum thyroiditis.*

   - **Menstrual Irregularities:** *Hormonal changes postpartum can cause irregular menstrual cycles.*

3. **Impact on Future Pregnancies**

   - ***Placenta Previa and Accreta:*** *Conditions such as placenta previa (where the placenta covers the cervix) and placenta accreta (where the placenta attaches too deeply into the uterine wall) are more common in women who have had previous C-sections.*

   - **Increased Risk of C-Sections:** *Women who have had one C-section are more likely to need a C-section in future pregnancies.*

Other Considerations

1. **Nutritional Deficiencies**
   - **Iron Deficiency:** *Blood loss during delivery can lead to anemia.*
   - **Calcium Deficiency:** *Pregnancy and breast-feeding can deplete calcium levels, affecting bone health.*

2. **Cardiovascular Health**
   - **Pre-eclampsia:** *Women who experienced pre-eclampsia (high blood pressure during pregnancy) have a higher risk of cardiovas-cular disease later in life.*

3. **Emotional Stress**
   - **Parenting Stress:** *The demands of caring for a newborn, especially with inadequate support, can lead to significant stress and affect overall well-being.*

So, as you see, pregnancy can have an immense impact on your health — I Googled it. After hearing about "The Baby" for the first time, I dug into it. Turns out, pre-existing health conditions might not magically vanish post-baby. I started to suspect a baby conspiracy here in my country, so I reached out to my friend, who has a teenage daughter, and asked her, "Jenny" (I changed the name) — so, Jenny, today I visited a doctor, and she advised me to give birth so my breast issues will be gone.

Jenny chuckled.

She said, "You know, Iryna, I visited my doctor recently too, had some minor kidney issues, and he asked me — did you give birth? I said — yes, why? And he said — I see, now I get why you have this issue. Giving birth can impact a woman's health severely, and not always in a good way (but of course, it depends)."

And I was like, "Okey-dokey, so now you say that curing my breast issue by giving birth might be a really bad idea?"

Jenny answered, laughing, "Moreover, it will give you tons of responsibilities, sleepless nights, numerous pains, and there is no guarantee that your issue will be important anymore (but it will definitely stay with you anyway)."

Yep, I thought so.

Don't get me wrong. I'm not against babies at all. They are cute. And if you want to have one — great!

But it wasn't my issue. I just wanted to feel a bit better, to have a normal life, and not to struggle with breast pain and cysts that were growing, changing, and scaring me to death. My body was scary now too; I couldn't control it anymore. (Yes, we can hardly control anything in our lives, but still.) I felt like it was letting me down. It was 2020, and I felt like I was descending deeper and deeper into this medical abyss. A place where you have to make check-ups every six months and live around the clock. Like — here's a check-up, cysts grew a bit, new ones emerged. So, here are your results: we have no idea what's happening with you, but see you in six months.

I came for help but wasn't getting any. In fact, now I felt like something was really wrong with me — or that I was losing my mind, a thought that haunted me ever since. I was really upset with the situation and decided to visit an oncologist. Oh yeah, that scary word made me numb, but I needed to hear what he had to say.

This doctor, very professional and attentive, checked me again, reviewed my ultrasound, asked me to do new blood tests and a hormone checkup, analyzed them attentively (including prolactin, which my gynecologists had been obsessively checking), and stated that I was okay. The cysts were not dangerous and sometimes happen to women. He also prescribed some herbal supplements meant to impact my prolactin and stress levels. And these supplements actually made me feel better — at least for the three months I was taking them.

Prolactin

Role:

- *Stimulates breast milk production after child-birth.*

- *Influences reproductive health and immune system function.*

That baby spell wasn't leaving my mind, though. All the gynecologists were pushing this "magic," but I didn't believe them anymore. So, I turned to the ultimate free source of information — the Internet. Because, seriously, you can't cure a condition with something as life-altering as giving birth, right? Right?... Or can you?

The Miracle of Hormones

During pregnancy, your body goes through a whirlwind of hormonal changes. These hormones, especially estrogen and progesterone, play a significant role in many aspects of your health. Sometimes, these hormonal shifts can have unexpected benefits.

Shrinking Cysts: A Possible Perk

Take breast cysts, for example. These are fluid-filled sacs that can develop in your breast tissue and are often harmless, but they can be uncomfortable. During pregnancy, the increased levels of hormones can sometimes cause these cysts to shrink or even disappear. It's like your body's way of doing a little spring cleaning while it's busy creating a new life.

Autoimmune Diseases: A Temporary Reprieve

For some women with autoimmune diseases, pregnancy can bring temporary relief. Conditions like rheumatoid arthritis and multiple sclerosis can go into remission during pregnancy. The exact reason isn't entirely understood, but it's thought that the immune system calms down a bit to prevent it from attacking the baby, which might also reduce its attack on the mother's body.

It's Not a Guarantee

While pregnancy can have these surprising benefits, it's not a guaranteed cure-all. In some cases, health issues can return after childbirth, sometimes with a vengeance. And there are other conditions that might worsen during pregnancy, so it's always important to keep your healthcare provider in the loop.

A Special Note on Breast Cancer

There's a myth that pregnancy can cure breast cancer. While hormonal changes can impact breast cysts, they do not cure breast cancer. Regular check-ups and screenings are crucial, regardless of pregnancy.

So, as you see, the breast issue really can be cured. But! No one can guarantee it. And that was a problem for me. I needed answers. I wanted to feel better. But it seemed that no one could help me with that.

I decided to find a new gynecologist, and I found one. We agreed that I would visit her every six months, we would do check-ups, and she wouldn't propose extreme methods. Thus, I decided to proceed with psychotherapy and find out if maybe there was something that bothered me. Perhaps I was fine, as the blood tests indicated, and all of this wasn't real, just a construct in my head.

Stress, maybe.

Or something else.

Chapter 5

There is a phrase that we don't know what we don't know. And it's true. In my situation, I had no idea what was happening, but I felt with every cell, every bone, and all my heart, that something was wrong.

I shared this nagging feeling with my doctors. They conducted thorough check-ups, scrutinized every angle, and ran numerous tests, yet found nothing serious. Despite their best efforts, they were essentially chasing their tails, focusing on "women's hormonal stuff." But I couldn't shake the feeling that it was something else entirely.

Each visit felt like a repeat episode of a medical drama, with no clear resolution in sight. The uncertainty gnawed at me. Was I imagining things? Was I overreacting? The medical professionals seemed to think so, but I trusted my instincts.

I'm not a doctor, but I do have extensive experience in academic research (I have a master's degree in management, and to earn it, I sometimes lived in the library). So, I started digging. If the doctors couldn't help me, maybe I could help myself.

The main task — and the most serious one — was to find the root cause of the problem. One evening, I retreated to my sanctuary: the kitchen. It's my favorite workspace, surrounded by plants and offering a view of breathtaking sunsets from my 10th-floor window. I took my notebook and prepared to do the hardest work in my life. Seriously, I've never felt this responsibility because my own health (and life) were on stake.

Image 5. Symptoms

By 2021, my symptoms had become a checklist of woes:

- Cysts
- A constant white noise in my head
- Persistent anxiety
- Difficulty falling asleep
- Relentless, intrusive thoughts
- Worsened allergy symptoms (flu-like issues, sore bones, and relentless tiredness)
- Occasional difficulty getting out of bed (though not every day)
- Low energy levels (I could barely remember what it felt like to have abundant energy, but I still maintained my 5-7 km daily walks)

I looked at the mental stuff — anxiety, and constant thoughts — and thought about it. It seemed like depression could be the cause. The thoughts, anxiety, and tiredness all fit. I talked about this with my therapist.

We discussed it together. I filled out a questionnaire and told her about my family problems and grief. Maybe all of that was causing my issues.

Depression

Depression is a mood disorder characterized by persistent feelings of sadness, hopelessness, and a lack of interest or pleasure in activities. It can affect how a person thinks, feels, and handles daily activities. Symptoms of depression can vary in severity and may include:

- *Persistent sad, anxious, or "empty" mood*
- *Feelings of hopelessness or pessimism*
- *Irritability*
- *Feelings of guilt, worthlessness, or helplessness*
- *Loss of interest or pleasure in hobbies and activities*
- *Decreased energy or fatigue*
- *Difficulty concentrating, remembering, or making decisions*
- *Difficulty sleeping, early-morning awakening, or oversleeping*
- *Appetite or weight changes*
- *Thoughts of death or suicide, or suicide attempts*
- *Physical symptoms such as headaches, digestive problems, or chronic pain that do not respond to treatment*

Depression can be caused by a variety of factors, including genetics, brain chemistry, personality, and life events.

Yes, I had some major life events — a death of a loved, a tough divorce, and some abuse. But I never thought about suicide. I've always been an active person who loves life, so it didn't seem like depression. But I was sad, felt a lot of guilt about the past, and was always anxious.

But it wasn't depression.

So, I was back at it, digging through information. The internet was my main source, but I stuck to scientific articles and reputable sources. I wasn't interested in gurus or miracle cures – I'm a pragmatist. I don't trust people who claim to cure everything with some mysterious, untested potion. This approach does make things tougher though — it narrows my options down to just medicine and science. But I'm okay with that.

I discovered that worm infestations can impact both our mood and physical health.

Worm infestations

Worm infestations, also known as helminthiasis, can cause a variety of symptoms depending on the type of worm and the severity of the infestation. Common symptoms include:

General Symptoms:

1. ***Digestive Issues:***
   - *Abdominal pain or discomfort*
   - *Diarrhea*
   - *Nausea and vomiting*
   - *Gas and bloating*
   - *Change in bowel habits*

2. ***Nutritional Deficiencies:***
   - *Weight loss*
   - *Loss of appetite*
   - *Malabsorption of nutrients leading to deficiencies (e.g., anemia due to hookworms)*
3. ***Fatigue and Weakness:***
   - *General feeling of tiredness*
   - *Weakness*
4. ***Skin Reactions:***
   - *Itchy rash*
   - *Allergic reactions*

I only had mental symptoms, no digestive issues, but rashes were popping up now and then. So, I decided to head to the lab and get checked.

Honestly, I felt a bit embarrassed and ridiculous. Here I was, a grown woman, getting tested for worms. It felt ironic. I wasn't eating dirt, I washed my food with soap, and I always kept my hands clean — yet here I was in this awkward situation. But, you know what? There's nothing weird or shameful about taking care of yourself. It's totally normal.

The tests came back clean.

"I thought so," I muttered to myself, diving even deeper into my research. Psychotherapy was helping as much as it could, but my symptoms just wouldn't vanish.

Then, out of nowhere, a memory jolted me — ten years ago, a tick had bitten me! Oh my, could it be Lyme disease?

I frantically googled the symptoms. Some of them matched – in fact, a lot of them did, and it was terrifying.

Chronic Lyme disease

Chronic Lyme disease, also known as Post-Treatment Lyme Disease Syndrome (PTLDS), can present a variety of symptoms that can persist for months or even years after initial treatment for Lyme disease. Symptoms can vary widely among individuals and may overlap with other conditions, making diagnosis challenging. Here are some common symptoms:

General Symptoms:

1. **Fatigue:**
   - *Persistent, severe tiredness that doesn't improve with rest*
   - *Exhaustion after minimal physical or mental activity*

2. **Musculoskeletal Pain:**
   - *Muscle aches*
   - *Joint pain and swelling, particularly in large joints like knees*
   - *Stiffness*

3. **Neurological Symptoms:**
   - *Headaches*
   - *Dizziness*
   - *Tingling, numbness, or burning sensations in extremities*

- *Facial palsy (loss of muscle tone or droop on one or both sides of the face)*
- *Memory problems and difficulty concentrating*
- *Mood changes, including depression and anxiety*

4. **Cognitive Difficulties:**
   - *"Brain fog"*
   - *Short-term memory issues*
   - *Difficulty finding words*
   - *Reduced ability to focus*

Cardiac Symptoms:

- *Palpitations*
- *Irregular heartbeats (arrhythmias)*
- *Chest pain*

Eye and Vision Symptoms:

- *Blurred vision*
- *Sensitivity to light (photophobia)*
- *Eye pain*

Digestive Symptoms:

- *Nausea*
- *Abdominal pain*
- *Diarrhea or constipation*

Other Symptoms:

- *Fever and chills*

- *Night sweats*
- *Unexplained weight loss or gain*
- *Swollen lymph nodes*

Psychological Symptoms:

- *Insomnia or other sleep disturbances*
- *Increased irritability*
- *Panic attacks*

Now, please don't laugh. There's a reason there's a song called "Never Google Your Symptoms" — it's true. The deeper you go into that rabbit hole, the worse you feel, and suddenly you find yourself with a bunch of new symptoms you never knew you had.

But I really had half of those symptoms, including strange joint pain in my fingers that came and went as it pleased.

So, I checked this idea. No, I didn't have Lyme disease. You can't have the chronic phase of something you never had in the first place. But I was desperate for answers. At this point, any explanation, even the most ridiculous, seemed possible.

Later, wild hypotheses popped into my head all the time. Partly because I'd read so much about different diseases, and partly because I was desperate to find any solution. I'd grab onto anything that wasn't even close to my symptoms, just to go and get another test done, only to find out it wasn't the problem.

And then there was that finger thing.

Chapter 6

The Mysterious Finger and The Huge Breast

When I was a kid, I spent summer vacations, about three glorious months, with my grandma and grandpa. Those were magical times in the village. I was outside almost all day, playing with friends, taking care of the garden, exploring the forest, swimming in the river, playing badminton, raising chickens, and just enjoying my life to the fullest.

It was also the time when I first woke up with a swollen thumb on my right hand. The thumb had doubled in size compared to its twin, and it hurt like hell. I was 11 or 12 at the time and went to show my granny this alarming sight. Long story short, she called grandpa, who came home from work and took me to the hospital. There, my poor thumb was X-rayed.

The thumb, though swollen, was declared healthy. The surgeon prescribed some ointment, and within a few days, the pain subsided, and the size returned to normal. The thumb was fine, and I moved on, forgetting all about it.

Later in life, this strange symptom would reappear unpredictably, affecting different fingers on both of my hands. Sometimes I assumed I had simply bumped a finger; the pain might vanish overnight, but other times, the finger would remain sore and immobile for days. I hadn't given it much thought until now. Amidst my intense health research, it hit me like a ton of bricks — this recurring issue was a symptom of multiple sclerosis.

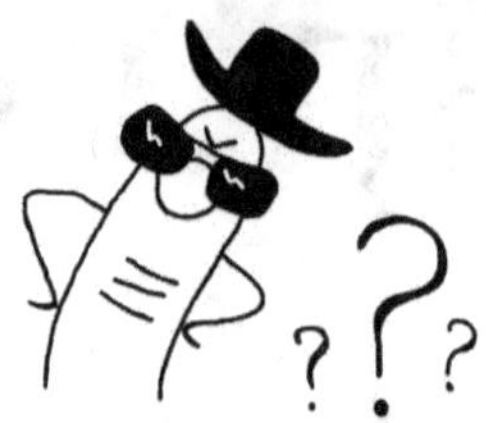

Image 6. The Finger

A-ha! — I thought and ran to the lab, because anxiety, fatigue, mood changes also were symptoms of this disease.

Have you ever noticed how many diseases share common symptoms? Especially when it comes to our mental state — our mood, anxiety, paranoia. It's as if our brain is desperately trying to warn us: "Hey, something's off! You need to address this!" It communicates in its own cryptic language, but we're often lost in translation.

I wish we had a better way to decode these signals.

What is Multiple Sclerosis?

Multiple Sclerosis (MS) is a chronic, often disabling disease that affects the central nervous system (CNS), which includes the brain and spinal cord. MS occurs when the immune system mistakenly attacks the protective sheath (myelin) that covers nerve fibers, leading to communication problems between the brain and the rest of the body. Eventually, the disease can cause the nerves themselves to deteriorate or become permanently damaged.

Symptoms:

Symptoms of MS vary widely among individuals and depend on the location and severity of the damage within the CNS. They can include:

1. ***Physical Symptoms:***

   - *Numbness or weakness in one or more limbs, typically on one side of the body at a time, or the legs and trunk.*

   - *Electric-shock sensations that occur with certain neck movements, especially bending the neck forward (Lhermitte sign).*

   - *Tremor, lack of coordination, or unsteady gait.*

   - *Partial or complete loss of vision, usually in one eye at a time, often with pain during eye movement (optic neuritis).*

   - *Prolonged double vision.*

   - *Blurry vision.*

2. ***Sensory Symptoms:***

   - *Tingling or pain in parts of your body.*

   - *Sensitivity to heat.*

   - *Spasticity (muscle stiffness and spasms).*

3. ***Cognitive Symptoms:***

   - *Slurred speech.*

   - *Fatigue.*

   - *Dizziness.*

- *Problems with bowel and bladder function.*
- *Cognitive changes including problems with memory, attention, and problem-solving.*

4. **Emotional Symptoms:**

- *Mood swings.*
- *Depression.*
- *Anxiety.*

My tests came back negative. By that point, I had lost all hope and was doing these tests more out of habit than expectation. I thought, "Well, if it works, it works. If not, I have to find a way to live my life and make it as decent as possible." I just wanted to wake up in the morning with a smile on my face.

I couldn't remember the last time I woke up with a smile. It was 2022, and I was stuck in a relentless cycle of medical check-ups every six months. I'd undergone another surgery for polyps in my uterus. I was perpetually tired and utterly exhausted. My breasts were swollen with cysts. Sleep eluded me. My moods swung like a pendulum; I was constantly irritated, anxious, and desperate. Happiness seemed like a distant memory.

And then, out of nowhere, a memory hit me like a freight train. Years ago, I woke up to find my right breast swollen to three times the size of my left. I was just a teenager, terrified out of my mind. The doctor who examined me said it was normal for someone my age. He explained that I was growing, my hormones were in overdrive, and this reaction, called mastopathy, was just part of the ride.

But now, being an adult, I felt that it wasn't normal at all.

Mastopathy

Mastopathy, also known as fibrocystic breast changes or fibrocystic breast disease, is a benign (non-cancerous) condition characterized by lumpy, painful breasts. It is a common condition that affects many women, particularly between the ages of 30 and 50. The changes are due to hormonal fluctuations, particularly those related to the menstrual cycle.

Symptoms:

The symptoms of mastopathy can vary from woman to woman, but common signs include:

1. ***Lumpy or Nodular Breast Tissue:***
   - *The presence of lumps or nodules that can feel tender or painful. These lumps are typically mobile and can change in size and tenderness throughout the menstrual cycle.*

2. ***Breast Pain or Tenderness:***
   - *Pain that can range from mild to severe. This pain often worsens before menstruation and improves afterward.*

3. ***Breast Swelling:***
   - *Swelling or a feeling of fullness in the breasts, which can also fluctuate with the menstrual cycle.*

4. ***Thickening of Breast Tissue:***
   - *Areas of thickened tissue that can be felt during a self-exam or by a healthcare provider.*

5. **Nipple Discharge:**

- *Sometimes, a clear, white, or slightly yellow nipple discharge can occur.*

Causes:

The exact cause of mastopathy is not fully understood, but it is believed to be related to hormonal fluctuations, particularly estrogen and progesterone. These hormones can cause the breast tissue to swell, leading to the formation of cysts and fibrous tissue.

I totally forgot about it, but now, when mastopathy had been my diagnosis for years, I began to wonder — what was really going on here? Why did my breast swell up so much back then? I couldn't just chalk it up to hormones; that situation was completely random and never happened again. My fingers, on the other hand, swelled more often but also quite randomly. Sometimes stress seemed to trigger it, sometimes not. It had started when I was a kid, so maybe the reason I felt so bad now lay somewhere in my childhood?

Again — the exact cause of mastopathy is unknown. Same with my symptoms — no one could explain what was going on, but there had to be a reason, I was sure of it.

But how can I figure out if it's a disease or not when I have no idea where to search or what to search for? It's like trying to solve a puzzle without knowing what the final picture looks like. The most important truth is, you don't know what you don't know.

But you must ask other people to find your answers.

Chapter 7

No matter how desperate I get, I always move towards my goal. Even when my willpower disappears, I keep thinking about it, and it really helps. Small steps always lead somewhere, even the tiniest ones.

So, I reached out to friends and family, asking for advice on

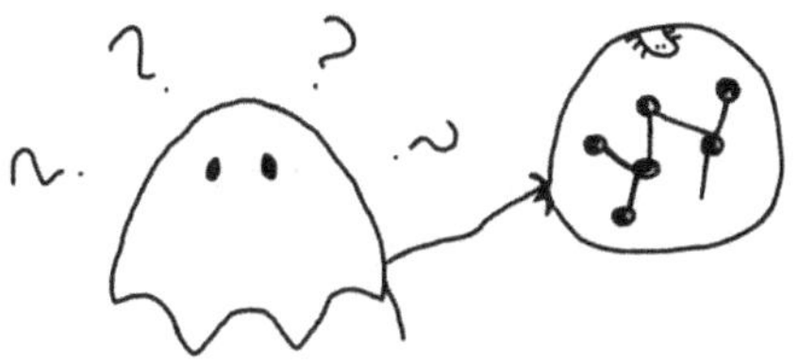

Image 7. Mysteries

whom I could visit for my issues. My mother-in-law recommended a new, young endocrinologist from their hospital. Thank goodness she's young, I thought. Women over 50 kept casting that baby spell on me, refusing to really listen. Eastern Europe, why, just why?

I came to this beautiful woman and said, "I'm nervous all the time. My reactions to everything are super sharp. I'm anxious. I have sleeping issues. I can do nothing about it. Can you help me?"

She replied, "Okay, let's check your blood pressure first."

A side note here: Throughout my exhausting journey, it

seemed like doctors didn't really believe I was sick. They acted as if I made everything up to gain their attention (I'm an adult with plenty of responsibilities — why would I do that?) or that I had minor issues, like a weak nervous system. They prescribed sedatives, calming pills, and advised me to go for massages or swimming. From their point of view, I was fine, as my blood tests were normal.

So, she checked my blood pressure (aside from the massive heartbeat and sweating, I also fear doctors, so it was a crazy mix and I was sure my blood pressure would be high). And voilà, my blood pressure was higher than normal. She looked at me and said, "Yes, you are nervous indeed."

I smiled. By the end of 2021, I was nervous all the time.

I have to go to the store? I'm nervous, I can't breathe, I'm sweating, and I don't want to go outside. Drive a car? Oh my god, no, not today, I just can't. Answer the phone?! No-no-no, no way. Meeting with friends? Gosh, maybe I'll just stay at home?! It's so calm and cozy here.

I have no idea how my boyfriend survived all that and didn't go crazy. I went crazy for sure. Because alongside being nervous, I was irritated. I snapped and yelled for minor reasons, and it was awful.

This doctor then asked me more questions. She asked, "Do you have some stressful events in your life? What is going on?" But aside from the COVID pandemic, everything was fine. I was spending a lot of time near the river, working, and starting to travel. Everything was fine, but I wasn't.

She then sent me to do more blood tests and also decided to check my cortisol levels.

Cortisol

Cortisol is a steroid hormone produced by the adrenal glands, which are located on top of each kidney. It is often referred to as the body's primary "stress hormone" because its levels rise in response to stress. Here are some key points about cortisol:

Role of Cortisol

1. ***Stress Response:*** *Cortisol plays a central role in the body's response to stress. When you perceive a threat or stressor, whether physical or psychological, the hypothalamus in the brain triggers the adrenal glands to release cortisol into the bloodstream. This initiates a cascade of physiological responses known as the "fight-or-flight" response, which prepares the body to deal with the stressor.*

2. ***Regulation of Metabolism:*** *Cortisol helps regulate metabolism by influencing how the body converts proteins, carbohydrates, and fats into energy. It increases blood sugar (glucose) levels by promoting gluconeogenesis (the production of glucose from non-carbohydrate sources like amino acids) and inhibiting insulin release from the pancreas.*

3. ***Immune Response:*** *Cortisol has anti-inflammatory properties and plays a role in modulating the immune response. It suppresses inflam-*

mation and reduces immune system activity, which helps to limit the body's inflammatory response to stress and injury.

4. **Other Functions:** Beyond its primary roles in stress response, metabolism, and immune function, cortisol also influences:

- *Blood Pressure: Cortisol helps regulate blood pressure by influencing vascular tone and fluid balance.*

- *Sleep-Wake Cycle: Cortisol levels typically follow a diurnal (daily) rhythm, with higher levels in the morning to help wake you up and lower levels in the evening to promote sleep.*

Effects of Chronic Cortisol Imbalance

- *Chronic Stress: Prolonged or chronic stress can lead to dysregulation of cortisol production, resulting in either chronically elevated or decreased levels. This imbalance can contribute to various health issues, including:*

  - *Metabolic Disorders: Such as insulin resistance, weight gain (especially around the abdomen), and increased risk of type 2 diabetes.*

  - *Immune Suppression: Chronic elevation of cortisol can suppress immune function, making individuals more susceptible to infections.*

- *Cardiovascular Problems: Elevated cortisol levels over time may contribute to hypertension (high blood pressure) and cardiovascular disease.*

- *Mental Health: Excess cortisol has been linked to anxiety, depression, and cognitive impairment.*

My cortisol levels were absolutely normal. She was surprised, thought for a moment, and then offered a piece of advice that genuinely saved my sanity during those times: "Incorporate some exercise before bed — cardio, dancing, whatever gets your heart pumping. It could help stabilize your state." That was the most impactful advice I ever received, and I pass it on to you, dear readers. Perhaps it will help someone out there drift into sleep more effortlessly.

She referred me to another specialist for an ultrasound of all my internal organs. They were mostly fine, but my pancreas showed some reactive changes that puzzled everyone. I had no major digestive issues, though I'd always had a low tolerance for large meals and fatty foods. The gastroenterologist advised me to maintain a healthy diet, avoid alcohol (which I already did), and be mindful of my eating habits.

My eating habits were pretty healthy — I didn't drink alcohol, I ate lots of fruits and vegetables, I chose high quality meat, fish, cheese, and reduced processed foods and fast food. What else could I reduce? I had no idea.

So, I found myself constantly shuttling between specialists: gynecologists, endocrinologists, my family doctor (who suggested cutting back on white bread), oncologist, and a psychotherapist, whom I've been visiting for years now, and who was a real blessing amidst the chaos.

Despite all these consultations and bills, none of them had a clue about what was truly wrong with me.

Chapter 8

In 2022, my state was even more disturbing — white noise in my head, sharp visceral reactions coursing through my body. Anxiety clung to me, triggering adrenaline surges at the slightest provocation — phone calls, work dilemmas, social interactions, casual conversations. Hell, I was constantly perspiring, my muscles tightened involuntarily, and scorching waves of heat swept through me every time someone approached me on the street.

It was terrifying, but I told myself — you have to live a normal life. Because, really, what else can you do? If this is how your body decides to operate with age (30+ is "the age," right?), you're getting older, and maybe it's your new baseline. So, pull yourself together and live your life. Maybe other people are grappling with this too? Look at them — they're happy, they're laughing. And so can you.

So, I lived my life. I juggled a mountain of work, maintained a private life, socialized with friends, and committed to fitness — wcight lifting, Pilates, yoga. I roamed outside for hours, trying to fill the dark void in my mind that was taking away all my joy — because my thoughts were racing like a high-speed chase, every minute, every second, and that mental cacophony grew louder and louder each day.

Physically, I felt myself becoming weaker too. Push-ups became a struggle, but I pushed through, convincing myself that exercise was good for me. My libido became lower than usual, and I started feeling paranoid. But, really, how can you even think about sex when you're constantly on high alert, tense, and agitated?! So, in my head, it made sense. It was my decline, and I accepted it.

I guess 2022 was the year I lost hope and decided to embrace my new identity. And I got used to it, especially because dancing and cardio helped. At least for a short while — after my workouts, there was a blissful silence in my head, and that was a true blessing.

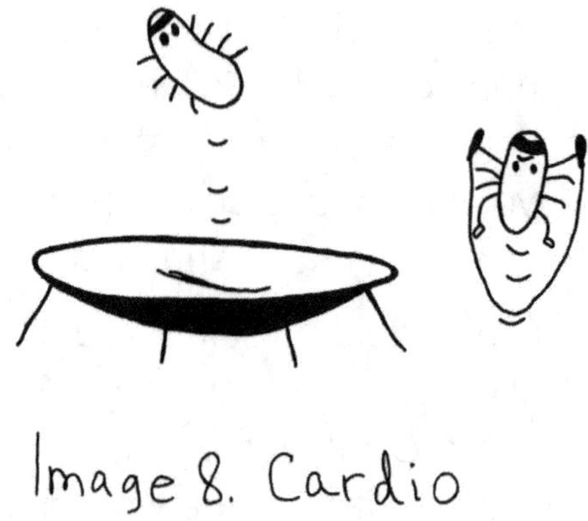

Image 8. Cardio

I was running, jumping, learned hip-hop dances on YouTube and played Nintendo dancing games. They made me really happy.

Cardio Training: Impact on Nervous System and Physical Body

Cardio training, also known as aerobic exercise, involves activities that increase the heart rate and promote cardiovascular health. Common forms of cardio training include running, cycling, swimming, and dancing. This type of exercise has numerous benefits for both the nervous system and the physical body.

Cardiovascular Health

Cardio training strengthens the heart muscle, enhancing its efficiency in pumping blood throughout the body. This results in improved circulation and a reduction in the workload on the heart. Regular aerobic exercise is associated with a lower risk of cardiovascular diseases, including heart disease, hypertension, and stroke.

Stress Reduction

Engaging in cardio training triggers the release of endorphins, which are hormones that promote a sense of well-being and reduce stress and anxiety. This biochemical response is often referred to as the "runner's high," and it can alleviate symptoms of depression and improve overall mood.

Cognitive Enhancement

Cardio training increases blood flow to the brain, supplying it with more oxygen and nutrients. This can lead to enhanced cognitive functions, including improved memory, attention, and problem-solving skills. Regular aerobic exercise has been shown to support brain health and may reduce the risk of cognitive decline as one ages.

Increased Energy Levels

Cardio exercise improves stamina and endurance by enhancing the body's ability to deliver oxygen to muscles. This results in higher energy levels and reduced fatigue during daily activities. Additionally, cardio training can improve sleep quality, contributing to better overall energy and alertness.

Immune System Support

Regular cardio workouts can strengthen the immune system by promoting good circulation. This enables immune cells to move more efficiently throughout the body, enhancing the body's ability to detect and fight off infections and illnesses.

Weight Management

Cardio training is an effective method for burning calories and managing weight. It boosts metabolism, allowing the body to burn calories more efficiently even after the workout has ended. When combined with a balanced diet, cardio exercise can help maintain a healthy weight and prevent obesity-related conditions.

Mood Improvement

The release of endorphins during cardio exercise can significantly elevate mood and provide a sense of well-being. This natural antidepressant effect can improve mental health and contribute to a positive outlook on life. The sense of achievement after completing a cardio workout can also boost self-confidence and motivation.

Longevity

Engaging in regular cardio exercise is linked to increased life expectancy. Aerobic activities help maintain healthy blood pressure and cholesterol levels, reduce the risk of chronic diseases, and promote overall physical health. This contributes to a longer, healthier life.

My endorphins were definitely doing their thing. Unfortunately, I can't say I made much headway with my physical shape. No matter how much I trained, I wasn't seeing significant muscle gains. My abs refused to tone up, and I stayed slender with a stubborn layer of fat around my stomach and legs. My body ached, and my breasts were more tender than usual, regardless of where I was in my cycle. Despite having checkups every six months, the cysts were only showing minor changes, but it seemed like those pesky processes in my body were slowing down.

Mental well-being remained unchanged, though. My gynecologist had stopped prescribing the herbal and other pills that had been helping to reduce the cysts. Those pills had been my lifeline for a couple of years. It's odd — they probably shouldn't have been effective, but I suspect their impact was a bit of a placebo miracle, a case of self-suggestion working its magic.

Chapter 9

The miracles of auto-suggestion

As you may remember, I refused to take hormonal pills. There was an inexplicable sense that something was off about them, a gut feeling I couldn't ignore. It was purely intuitive, clashing with conventional wisdom. Doctors were insistent on oral contraceptives, and there was plenty of evidence suggesting these could help dissolve breast cysts. Yet, I couldn't buy into it. My symptoms seemed so misaligned with their claims.

Then there were the blood tests. It felt strange to take medication when my hormone levels were perfectly normal, don't you think? The questions and doubts were tormenting me. I was already feeling ill, under intense pressure from doctors warning of worsening conditions and possible future surgeries. But in the end, my intuition was right. I was correct to trust my instincts.

Trust yourself. Always. When you notice contradictions, or when, despite having poured over countless sources of information, you sense that something crucial is missing from the puzzle — trust that feeling. Yes, there are contradictions. Yes, your intuition is valid. You simply don't know what you don't know.

Hormonal Therapy

Oral Contraceptives: *Oral contraceptives, commonly known as birth control pills, are sometimes prescribed to manage breast cysts. These pills regulate hormonal fluctuations during the menstrual cycle, which can reduce the development and recurrence of cysts. By stabilizing hormone levels, oral contraceptives can help minimize the formation of cysts and the discomfort they cause.*

Anti-inflammatory Medications

Nonsteroidal Anti-inflammatory Drugs (NSAIDs): *NSAIDs, such as ibuprofen, are commonly used to relieve pain and inflammation associated with breast cysts. While they do not directly reduce cyst size, they can alleviate discomfort and improve quality of life for women experiencing cyst-related pain.*

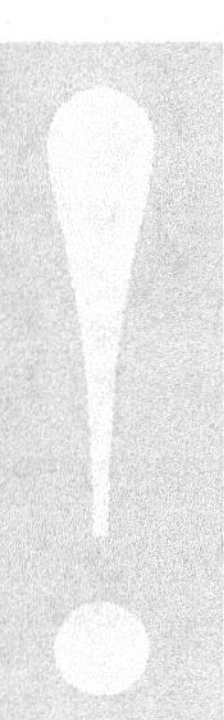

Seeing my refusal to take oral contraceptives, my doctors opted for a third approach. Different doctors, over various time periods, recommended the same herbal remedies. Clearly, these remedies had helped others, which is why I decided to give them a shot. I was willing to try anything and go anywhere if it meant finding answers to my questions — Why is this happening? What am I doing wrong? How can I put an end to this? But such a place didn't exist at that time.

The chosen remedy was chasteberry extract, combined with a synthetic substance called epigalin. This chasteberry extract acted on me like a mild antidepressant — it improved my mental state, reduced my irritation, and brought me a sense of strength and better sleep.

Chasteberry Extract for Women's Hormonal Issues

Chasteberry, also known as Vitex agnus-castus, is a fruit from the chaste tree native to the Mediterranean region and Asia. It has been used for centuries in herbal medicine to address various women's health issues, particularly those related to hormonal imbalances. The extract of chasteberry is derived from its dried fruit and is available in various forms, including capsules, tinctures, and teas.

Mechanism of Action

Chasteberry is believed to influence the pituitary gland, which in turn affects the production of several hormones. The exact mechanism is not fully understood, but it is thought to increase the release of luteinizing hormone (LH) while mildly inhibiting the release of follicle-stimulating hormone (FSH). This can lead to an increase in progesterone production and a balancing effect on estrogen and progesterone levels in the body.

Uses and Benefits

1. **Premenstrual Syndrome (PMS):** *Chasteberry is commonly used to alleviate symptoms of PMS, such as breast tenderness, mood swings, irritability, and headaches. Several studies have shown that women taking chasteberry extract report a reduction in these symptoms, likely due to its hormone-regulating effects.*

2. **Premenstrual Dysphoric Disorder (PMDD):** *For women with PMDD, a severe form of PMS, chasteberry can also provide relief. Its ability to balance hormones may help mitigate the extreme mood disturbances and physical symptoms associated with this condition.*

3. **Irregular Menstrual Cycles:** *Women with irregular menstrual cycles, whether due to hormonal imbalances, polycystic ovary syndrome (PCOS), or other factors, may benefit from chasteberry. By normalizing the production of reproductive hormones, it can help regulate the menstrual cycle and promote more predictable periods.*

4. **Menopausal Symptoms:** *Although less common, chasteberry is sometimes used to ease menopausal symptoms. Its effects on hormone regulation can help reduce hot flashes, night sweats, and mood changes during menopause.*

5. **Fertility Issues:** *Chasteberry has been used to address fertility issues related to hormonal imbalances. By promoting the regularity of the menstrual cycle and supporting progesterone levels, it can enhance ovulation and improve the chances of conception for some women.*

The maximum duration for which I took those pills was six months. The cysts didn't vanish, but I was able to live a more normal life than before. My breasts felt better, and even my mood improved significantly. I intermittently took the pills from 2020 to 2022, but over time, I noticed that the initial magical effect began to wane, gradually but steadily.

Reflecting on those times now, I'm astounded by the power of faith and auto-suggestion. It's remarkable — you're treating the wrong issue, yet the medication still seems to work and improve how you feel, at least for a few months. It's incredible how we can endure various creepy things, live with persistent anxiety, and still manage to create small miracles for ourselves.

What is Auto-Suggestion?

Auto-suggestion involves the deliberate practice of planting specific ideas or beliefs into one's mind with the intention of altering perceptions, attitudes, or behaviors. It is based on the principle that the subconscious mind can be influenced by repetitive positive statements, which can lead to changes in thought patterns and, ultimately, behavior. This technique is widely used in self-help, personal development, and therapeutic settings.

Miracles of Auto-Suggestion

1. ***Enhanced Self-Confidence:***

   - *By repeatedly affirming positive statements about oneself, individuals can boost their self-esteem and confidence. This can lead to improved performance in various areas, such as public speaking, sports, or career advancement.*

2. ***Improved Health:***

   - *Auto-suggestion can play a significant role in promoting better health. Affirmations focused on wellness, healing, and vitality can help reduce stress, improve immune function, and accelerate recovery from illness.*

3. ***Behavioral Changes:***

   - *This technique can aid in overcoming negative habits and adopting positive ones. For instance, affirmations like "I am free from smoking" or "I choose healthy foods" can support efforts to quit smoking or improve diet.*

4. ***Emotional Well-being:***

   - *Regular use of positive affirmations can help manage emotions, reduce anxiety, and alleviate depression. Statements such as "I am calm and centered" or "I release all negative thoughts" can contribute to emotional stability.*

5. ***Achieving Goals:***

   - *Self-suggestion can enhance motivation and focus, helping individuals stay committed to their goals. Affirmations like "I am dedicated to my success" or "I achieve my goals with determination" can drive persistence and effort.*

6. **Stress Reduction:**

   - *By focusing on calming and reassuring affirmations, individuals can manage stress more effectively. Statements such as "I am at peace" or "I handle challenges with ease" can foster a sense of tranquility.*

Scientific Basis

While auto-suggestion may sound like a mystical concept, it has roots in psychological theories and practices. Cognitive-behavioral therapy (CBT), for example, uses similar principles by encouraging individuals to challenge and change negative thought patterns. The placebo effect also demonstrates the power of the mind in influencing physical health outcomes, further supporting the idea that what we believe can significantly impact our reality.

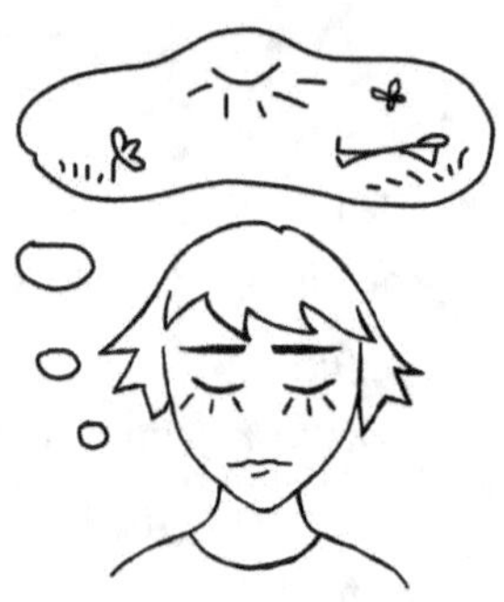

Image 9. Thoughts

It's not like I was deliberately practicing auto-suggestion or using it as a technique. Not at all. I simply had faith in medicine and trusted my doctors, even though they were more like observers than active helpers.

I constantly reassured myself, soothing my anxious inner child with promises that everything would be okay, that I would get better, that the medication would work, and one day I'd wake up feeling fantastic again. And, you know what? I did feel better and genuinely believed it was the right path for me. Maybe it was placebo – who's to say? But who knows. The human body is such a complex system, and we still don't fully understand how it all works when it comes to diseases, recovery, and the impact of our thoughts.

Now that I see the whole picture, I'm both amazed and astonished that my body managed to function for so long while struggling so much. It's incredible that it continued to operate, and even improved with medications that eased some of the symptoms. The whole system responded with positive changes. It's truly remarkable. Our bodies are amazing.

The positive effects were most noticeable each time I took the pills, especially during the first two months of treatment. However, after the third month, despite taking them intermittently over two years, I observed a constant, subtle decline. My anxiety made a comeback, like an old friend saying, "Hello again, I'm here to stay. Embrace me, because I'm not going anywhere."

In 2023, things took a turn for the worse. My doctors stopped prescribing the pills, insisting I was fine and admitting they had no idea why the polyps were coming back, why my breasts hurt, or why my body was out of sorts. I still recall my gynecologist – whether the 5th or 6th, I can't quite remember – trying to reassure me after she discovered I needed surgery again (and an ASAP breast ultrasound every three months). She said, "I have a patient with a similar issue, and the only state she's okay in is pregnancy."

Aside from being angry, I was also deeply sad. Being a woman in Eastern Europe can be incredibly draining, I must admit. It often feels like you're not fully human without children, as if you don't have the right to feel good or be healthy. But I tried not to dwell on that. As an adult, I know what I need, regardless of what others say. It's called determination, and it's part of the resilient me who endured that childhood medical nightmare.

I thought, "Wow, that's fantastic. Doctor, can you help me? No! But hey, maybe if you get pregnant, you'll feel better. Who knows? We're clueless. But here's a baby spell for you!"

That's when I finally lost all hope.

Chapter 10

Where the resilience comes from?

As a kid, I was sick nearly all the time. Every spring brought a new set of problems — coughs, high fevers, or severe sinusitis. I had chickenpox, numerous flus, and pneumonias. Ask me about any illness, and I can probably share a story. Thankfully, I was vaccinated against a lot of diseases, so I wasn't as sick as I might have been otherwise.

I dealt with pancreas issues and food poisoning, gallbladder problems, and a few drug allergies (the only allergies diagnosed back then). I experienced a slew of symptoms and endured a lot of suffering.

I love spring, but every March, I had this nagging feeling that something bad was just around the corner. Sure enough, come April or May, on a sunny morning, I'd find myself with a high fever, a cough, and struggling to breathe through my nose. I'd feel utterly miserable, leading my parents to rush me to the hospital, and the cycle of medical procedures would begin anew. The nose-cleaning procedures were the worst — they were excruciatingly painful and made breathing feel like inhaling fire. It was the post-Soviet approach to medicine, harsh and inhumane, and no one ever seemed to care about how I felt afterward.

I was in constant pain during the spring months, but I had no idea that something as simple as a small white pill called an "antihistamine" could make a difference. Kids aren't supposed to know about these things, after all. So, like a small but brave soldier, I endured, desperately trying to navigate the troubles that life, the gods, or destiny — whatever you want to call it — threw my way. Every morning, I'd tell myself that the pain would pass and I'd eventually get better.

But the next year, it all started over again.

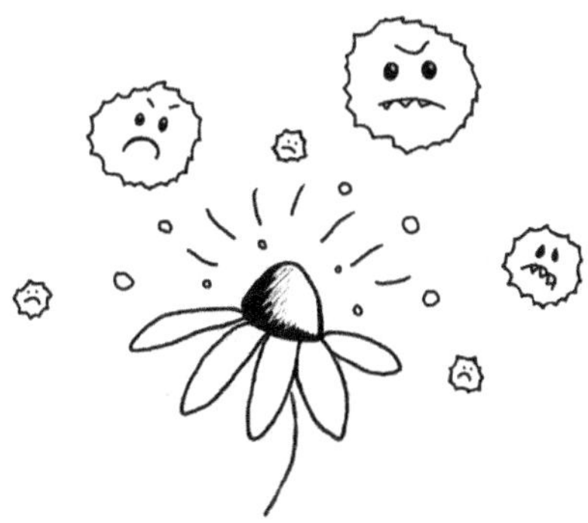

Image 10. Pollen

Add in countless food poisonings and persistent pancreas pain, and it felt like the cycle would never end.

You might wonder — hadn't anyone questioned your diet or checked for allergies with all this spring stuff going on? Nope, neither the doctors nor my parents seemed particularly concerned about these issues. They just treated the symptoms and repeated the mantra, "It's kids; they get sick. Often."

By my 20s, I had improved; all symptoms were gone except for a relentless cough that felt like it was tearing apart my lungs, leaving me limp and exhausted. The doctors I visited would listen to my lungs and bronchi, prescribe pills, and that was about it. It wasn't until I was 28 that a fantastic otolaryngologist — who had over 40 years of experience — finally identified my spring allergies. It took her just three minutes to reach the correct diagnosis. Three minutes. As a kid, no one ever told me this. I had suffered in complete silence. My parents were so busy with making a living that they completely overlooked my needs. I was left to face this alone — frustrated and scared. It was then, as a child, that I decided I'd have to manage on my own. I'd live a normal life despite the pain and fear. If no one else could help me, then I would! My body might be weak, but there are plenty of people with weak bodies living their best lives.

I think I was born resilient — strong and joyful, no matter the circumstances. To me, life felt magical and endless, brimming with beauty, wonderful people, and nature. Despite my physical issues, I was happy. I excelled in physical training at university, always active and full of energy. It seemed like nothing could shatter my resilience.

By the end of 2022, it felt like my star team of superheroes — my body and I — had become estranged. My body was letting me down, and the joy I once found in life was slipping away. I hardly ever smiled, and every morning felt like a struggle — wondering, "Why should I even get up if this day won't be any better?" My breasts ached even more, and I had little desire to interact with people. I mostly confined myself to working or watching films on my laptop.

I have no idea how my boyfriend managed to stick around. I was so sick and tired of myself (and him) that I felt like I'd become a crazy old cat lady, shouting and cursing like a sailor. Life was unbearable, and I seriously considered leaving him to be alone because only when I was by myself could I somewhat manage the irritation and anxiety. Being around people was impossible; they needed my attention, and I was so mentally preoccupied that I couldn't focus on them.

I'm not sure how I managed to maintain relationships with my friends — it was probably just sheer willpower, a resilience I'd built up from early years. My anxious side wanted to burn everything down and run away. But how do you escape when it's you who's in charge?

Yet, despite it all, I couldn't forget the suffering from my childhood and was determined not to repeat it. I was set on finding the reason and the solution. I was ready to crawl toward it, think about it, and uncover it in the end.

You might wonder why I didn't ask for help. That's why this book exists — I did ask. But people weren't really listening. Traditional medicine focused on treating individual organs, and I hadn't found anyone who viewed me as a whole system. Something was clearly off, but there was no mechanic to fix the broken parts of me.

Plus, here's an intriguing phenomenon: if you boil a frog slowly, it won't notice the danger until it's too late.

The Metaphor

The metaphor itself is derived from the story that if a frog is placed in boiling water, it will immediately jump out to escape the danger. However, if the frog is placed in cold water that is gradually heated, it will not perceive the gradual increase in temperature and will eventually be boiled alive. While the literal truth of this experiment is debated, the metaphor serves as a powerful illustration of how gradual change can lead to unnoticed, potentially harmful outcomes.

Psychological Practice

In psychological terms, "boil the frog slowly" can be understood in various contexts:

1. **Adaptation to Negative Situations:**

   - Individuals might gradually adapt to increasingly negative circumstances without realizing the full extent of the changes. This can occur in abusive relationships, toxic work environments, or unhealthy habits. The gradual increase in negativity makes it harder for individuals to recognize and react to the worsening situation.

2. **Behavioral Change:**

   - Gradual, small changes are introduced to modify behavior over time. For instance, in cognitive-behavioral therapy, incremental steps are used to address phobias or anxiety, making the change less overwhelming and more manageable.

3. **Persuasion and Influence:**

   - Marketers, leaders, or influencers might use this approach to slowly shift attitudes or behaviors. By introducing small changes or ideas progressively, they can lead individuals to adopt new beliefs or habits without resistance.

4. ***Social and Cultural Shifts:***

   - *Societal norms and values can shift slowly over time through incremental changes. What might be considered unacceptable or unusual at one point can become normalized through gradual acceptance and integration.*

Real-World Examples

1. ***Abusive Relationships:***

   - *An abusive partner might start with minor controlling behaviors that escalate over time. The victim may not recognize the severity of the abuse until it has significantly impacted their well-being and freedom.*

2. ***Work Environment:***

   - *A workplace might gradually increase demands on employees, such as longer hours or increased workloads, without corresponding rewards or recognition. Over time, employees may experience burnout without realizing how significantly their work conditions have deteriorated.*

3. ***Health and Lifestyle:***

   - *Poor dietary habits, lack of exercise, or increasing stress can gradually lead to significant health issues. Individuals might not notice the gradual decline in their health until they face serious consequences like obesity, heart disease, or mental health disorders.*

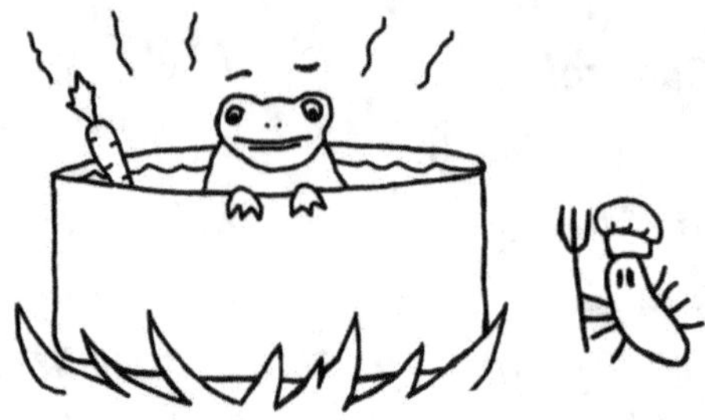

Image 11. Boiling the frog

I was that frog. The changes in my physical and mental state were gradual and slow, but the result I faced in December 2022 was terrifying. One day, I suddenly realized I couldn't even stand listening to my boyfriend — his voice was grating, and our relationship issues felt overwhelming. It hit me out of nowhere; I had this alarm ringing in my brain and thought, "THIS is not normal." My constant anxiety had become a sort of background noise, something I was used to, even if it was overwhelming. But this new level of distress was much more alarming.

I freaked out and decided to see a psychiatrist.

Note: I have no idea how others handle these situations. I chose to consult a mental health specialist because I knew they dealt with issues like mine. Despite my general disappointment with doctors and medicine, I recognized that simple yoga or mindfulness wouldn't cut it, as they hadn't helped before. The same went for psychotherapy.

Moreover, by the end of 2022, I had been in psychotherapy for four years and had resolved almost all of my issues, including childhood trauma, divorce, and other sources of extreme unhappiness. I wanted to feel normal or even joyful, but instead,

I was stressed out and profoundly sick. It wasn't just a mental issue, I concluded; there must have been something off in my brain chemistry (that's how I was thinking at the time), because the hormones — at least the ones doctors were checking — were okay.

That's how I ended up in the office of this kind and understanding psychiatrist. I'd never been to such an appointment before, so I had no idea how to behave. In fact, I was so nervous that when she asked me why I decided to come, I blurted out:

"Something is wrong with me. I'm incredibly anxious, can't sleep properly, am exhausted from my own thoughts, and my relationships are falling apart. Doctors say my hormones are fine, but I'm not. Maybe it's depression or something worse. I can't stop my racing thoughts."

Long story short, she asked about my life, my relationships, my progress in psychotherapy, and all my symptoms. We discovered that I was stuck in certain thought patterns that were preventing me from moving forward. These were issues we hadn't previously discussed, but they were quietly eroding my mental well-being from within. Relationships are tough, and my constant urge to escape wasn't just a personal quirk—it was influenced by an unknown illness that was impacting me in ways I hadn't fully grasped.

She said, "I think you have neurosis. I'll prescribe you some mild calming pills, and then we'll see how things go. I don't want to prescribe antidepressants because I don't believe you have classic depression."

In the end, she was right — I didn't have ordinary depression. What I was experiencing was something entirely different.

Neurosis

Neurosis is a class of functional mental disorders involving chronic distress but neither delusions nor hallucinations. It is primarily characterized by anxiety, depression, or other feelings of unhappiness or distress that are out of proportion to the circumstances of a person's life but without a radical loss of touch with reality. This term was replaced with the "anxiety disorders" category in 1980.

Causes

Anxiety disorder can result from a combination of factors:

- **Genetic Predisposition:** *A family history of anxiety or depressive disorders can increase the likelihood of developing this disorder.*

- **Biological Factors***: Imbalances in neurotransmitters such as serotonin and dopamine can contribute to neurotic symptoms.*

- **Environmental Stressors:** *Traumatic events, chronic stress, and significant life changes can trigger or exacerbate neurotic conditions.*

- **Psychological Factors:** *Early childhood experiences, personality traits, and learned behaviors can influence the development of anxiety disorders.*

Symptoms

Symptoms may vary depending on the specific disorder but commonly include:

- **Emotional Symptoms:** *Persistent sadness, anxiety, irritability, or feelings of inadequacy.*

- **Cognitive Symptoms:** *Recurrent, unwanted thoughts, excessive worry, difficulty concentrating.*

- **Physical Symptoms:** *Fatigue, sleep disturbances, muscle tension, and somatic complaints without a medical cause.*

- **Behavioral Symptoms:** *Avoidance of feared situations, compulsive behaviors, social withdrawal.*

Anxiety disorder? That sounded reasonable. I Googled it, did my own research, and then started the treatment. I even rented a flat and decided to live on my own for a month or two, which my boyfriend agreed might help us address our issues more effectively.

Plus, I was desperate for silence. I needed to be alone.

After a few weeks of this new setup, I felt much better mentally. But something interesting happened with those pills. I never thought self-hypnosis was real because I didn't really believe in it, yet here we were. Every treatment I'd had over the past 10 years seemed to help — I felt better, my nervous system was calmer (though not entirely), and my body felt lighter and stronger. But after about two months, everything started to revert to its previous (or even worse) state, slowly but surely.

The same thing happened with neurosis: I felt better, I moved back in with my boyfriend, slept more soundly, and became more active overall. The pills helped, and I continued with my life.

Of course, I wasn't 100% fine (when was I ever?), but my mornings weren't unbearable. We resolved our issues, and my neurosis seemed to vanish. But then, two months later, the anxiety crept back in. It doesn't mean I didn't have anxiety while dealing with neurosis — I did. It was with me constantly, but it was… muted? Weaker? It felt like there was a wall between me and my anxiety. I experienced a similar state when I was taking other medications prescribed to me over the years.

In May 2023, I went for a checkup and found out that while the polyps were gone, my breast cysts had grown larger. Summer 2023 was a challenging time for me. I struggled with insomnia, anxiety, and irritability. Hot flashes would rush through my body, leaving me sweating and nervous, my thoughts racing uncontrollably. Long walks didn't help much, but swimming did, so I spent 4-5 hours daily at the beach and in the river, seeking solace in the water.

By October 2023, the polyps were back. My breasts were sore again, and despite my prolactin levels being normal, I was told I needed another surgery.

I came home from the hospital and locked myself in my office. I cried and cried, unable to stop. My mind was racing with thoughts about the future — could I endure this again next year? Or for ten years in a row? Would I be able to withstand this state without breaking down completely after fifteen more years of such a life? I had no answers. It became painfully clear that I needed to do something, but the only solution that came to mind was escape. Move to another country. Run.

But you can't run from yourself, right?

Chapter 11

When you friends come to rescue

I had my surgery in January 2024. The months from October to January were a time I chose to spend indulging in relaxation and pleasure, luxuries I couldn't afford before because I was always running and grinding, trying to silence my anxiety and pretend I was fine. I had plenty of work to do, and I did it excellently. But at what cost? I felt like I was slowly dying, so I decided to take care of myself this time. No matter what the future held, I planned to relax.

I partied with my friends, surrounded myself with positive vibes, and enjoyed good movies, books, and my favorite foods (including homemade yogurts with fresh berries, of course). I embraced gardening, and when the first snow covered our village fields, I took to sledging.

All that was a good distraction. I have great memories from that time.

I was also ready to meet this next surgery and whatever came next like a small but courageous hobbit, heading to face Sauron and somehow survive this rendezvous.

At the end of 2023, I visited my dentist for my annual check-up. Kate took a look at my teeth and asked, "Are you eating well?" I responded, "Yeah, I eat pretty healthily." She nodded, noting that she'd followed me on Instagram for a while and had seen my daily food posts — fruits, berries, veggies, dairy, meat, fish, pizza, and burgers (because seriously, nothing beats pizza and burgers — well, maybe homemade gran's varenyky and pies).

But there was one thing that had been bugging me for a couple of months: my teeth were insanely sensitive. Even cold water felt sharp, hot food was uncomfortable, and sour stuff was off-limits. I'd never had this kind of tooth sensitivity before, and it had me worried.

Kate advised me to be more cautious with my dental care and recommended using an irrigator.

What is teeth sensitivity?

Teeth sensitivity, also known as dentin hypersensitivity, occurs when the protective layers of your teeth are compromised. This exposes the inner layer called dentin, which has tiny tubules leading to the tooth's nerve center. When these tubules are exposed to hot, cold, sweet, or acidic foods, or even a gust of cold air, it can cause a painful sensation.

Causes of Teeth Sensitivity:

1. ***Tooth Decay and Cavities:*** *These can create openings in the enamel, exposing the dentin.*

2. ***Gum Recession:*** *As gums pull back, they expose the root surfaces of the teeth, which are not protected by enamel.*

3. ***Brushing Too Hard:*** *Overzealous brushing can wear down enamel and expose dentin.*

4. ***Grinding Teeth:*** *Also known as bruxism, grinding can wear away enamel over time.*

5. ***Dental Procedures:*** *Teeth can be temporarily sensitive after procedures like fillings, crowns, or teeth whitening.*

6. **Acidic Foods and Drinks:** *Consuming a lot of acidic foods and beverages can erode enamel.*

7. **Cracked Teeth:** *Cracks can reach down to the dentin, leading to sensitivity.*

8. **Plaque Buildup:** *A heavy buildup of plaque can cause sensitivity.*

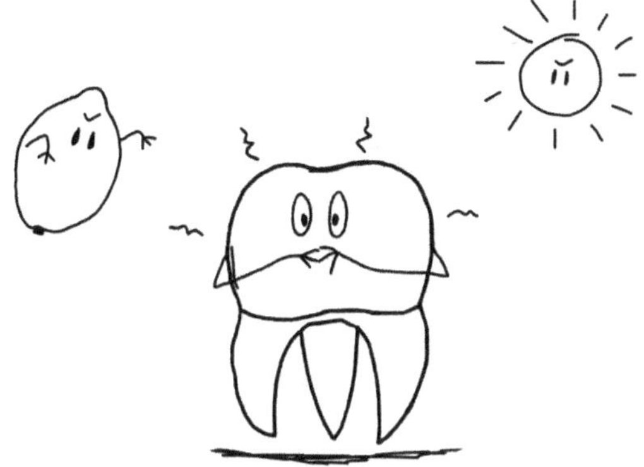

Image 12. The Tooth

Naturally, I Googled it and found that most of the usual causes didn't fit my situation — I wasn't brushing too hard, had regular check-ups, addressed all minor issues, and generally took good care of my teeth.

But one thought kept nagging at me: could it be related to my diet? Was it something I was eating? (I'd been consuming a lot of blueberries that autumn.) Or could it be a mix of factors? How was I supposed to pinpoint them?

My dentist didn't have an explanation, so I pushed that theory aside and tried to live life to the fullest. However, I could only fall asleep with the help of melatonin and herbal calming pills, and my sweating issues were getting worse. I was working out more, but saw zero results — just the usual morning soreness indicating that my muscles had been working hard.

The food issue was on my mind constantly. I'd never considered food allergies before.

I also realized something else — this strange condition was making me careless, out of touch, and insecure. I kept thinking about my diet, but in 2023, I didn't take any action to visit an allergy clinic and check for food allergies. I just waited for months, until the surgery, doing nothing in between.

This wasn't me; it was the disease. I didn't even recognize myself in that version of me anymore.

Chapter 12

The hardest part for me was coming to terms with the fact that I was truly alone. Sure, I had friends and family who supported me, but they couldn't fully grasp what was happening inside my body and mind. I'd felt isolated as a kid in the hospital, dealing with allergies that weren't properly addressed.

But this adult loneliness felt different.

As an adult, you're juggling responsibilities — work, people, kids, pets, and the never-ending task of putting groceries on the table. You've got to plan for the future and keep moving forward. You can't just hit pause and let your life unravel.

When life becomes overwhelming, and it feels like no one truly understands your struggle, when every diagnosis seems off, doctors insist you're fine, and you're staring at an impenetrable wall that feels like it might be the end — because you've run out of strength to push and climb — this is when loneliness wraps around you like a heavy shroud. It envelops you and isolates you from the world. Movement and breath become impossible as you struggle to break free, but it's futile. For me, this state wasn't quiet either — my thoughts piled up like a chaotic symphony of discordant sounds, a frenzy of madness in my mind. I battled them relentlessly, but they fought back with equal ferocity. All my childhood issues, work frustrations, relationship problems — they roared in my ears around the clock. Even my dreams grew more intense and stressful, as if all my unresolved traumas were staging a "hi" from the shadows. I woke up almost every night with my heart racing. I tried to juggle my daily roles as a gardener, girlfriend, daughter, sister, and friend, but I kept failing.

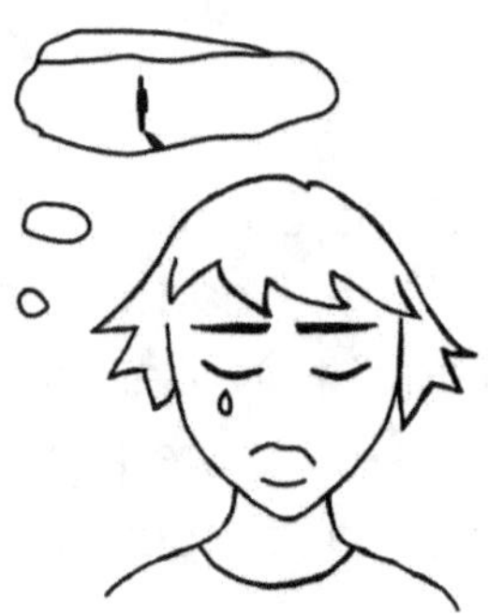

Image 13. Loneliness

You need to understand that this state didn't hit me all at once (if it had, I would have rushed to the clinic immediately). It built up gradually — I'd been simmering in anxiety for years, and the pressure was mounting slowly, day by day. But the moment of realizing my dire situation was abrupt. Bam — there I was, crying in my office, unable to stop, overwhelmed by a life that felt intolerable, with no idea of what was happening or what steps to take next.

I always believed that in moments like these, you need to summon your inner strength. It's when your internal fortitude has to rise up and save you — ancient forces that stir within your heart. My own experience taught me that neither God, external mystical forces, Greek gods, nor forest witches are coming to your rescue. No one's observing your struggle from above. The gods can't save you.

But people can.

I reached a point where I felt I couldn't go on any longer. I'd been rescuing myself for so long and holding on so tightly that I couldn't remember the last time I just relaxed with a glass of lemonade, lost in thought. I couldn't unwind, silence my racing thoughts, or ease the constant anxiety. I was completely spent, and all that remained of me was a façade — a mask I wore, while beneath it, I was crying and screaming.

It wasn't depression in the conventional sense. That's why my psychiatrist didn't prescribe antidepressants, and she was right. At that point in my life, I seriously considered two options: either burn my existing life to the ground (because maybe, just maybe, it was the root of my problems and all of this was just collateral damage) and start fresh in a new country with new people — or swim out into the river, so far that coming back would be impossible, given my poor swimming skills. Honestly, I couldn't even swim "far away" because I was terrified of deep water. I needed to feel the ground beneath my feet at all times.

When I heard these thoughts in my own mind, I was terrified. This was completely out of character, and IT WASN'T ME speaking. It was something else — my disease manifesting itself.

I had no idea what to do. I thought I would never escape this dark void. Then, out of nowhere, my friend Alyona came to the rescue — magically and unexpectedly.

Alyona knew all about my surgeries, and she was deeply into holistic medicine, supplements, and spiritual journeys (a bit woo-woo, yes, but we had plenty to talk about), alongside conventional medicine.

Just as I was contemplating "swimming far away," two or three weeks before my surgery, Alyona sent me a video. An Armenian doctor was discussing dairy and its negative impact on women's health.

Negative Effects of Dairy on Women's Health

While dairy products like milk, cheese, and yogurt are often touted for their nutritional benefits, including calcium and vitamin D, some women may experience negative health effects from consuming dairy. Here's a look at some potential downsides:

1. **Lactose Intolerance:**

   - **What It Is:** *Lactose intolerance is the inability to properly digest lactose, the sugar found in milk and dairy products.*

   - **Symptoms:** *Bloating, gas, diarrhea, and abdominal pain after consuming dairy.*

   - **Prevalence:** *It's more common in certain ethnic groups, including African American, Asian, and Hispanic women.*

2. **Allergies:**

   - **What It Is:** *A dairy allergy involves the immune system reacting to proteins found in milk, such as casein and whey.*

   - **Symptoms:** *Hives, wheezing, digestive issues, and in severe cases, anaphylaxis.*

   - **Management:** *Complete avoidance of dairy products is usually necessary for those with a true allergy.*

3. **Hormonal Imbalance:**

   - **What It Is:** *Some studies suggest that the hormones present in dairy products, especially* those derived from pregnant cows, might influence human hormone levels.

- **Potential Effects:** Acne, menstrual irregularities, and potentially an increased risk of hormone-related cancers, though research is ongoing and not yet conclusive.

4. **Digestive Issues:**

- **What It Is:** Even women without lactose intolerance can sometimes experience digestive discomfort from dairy.

- **Symptoms:** Gas, bloating, and cramps.

- **Possible Causes:** High-fat content in certain dairy products or individual sensitivities.

5. **Bone Health Controversy:**

- **What It Is:** While dairy is promoted for bone health due to its calcium content, some research suggests high dairy consumption may not necessarily lead to stronger bones.

- **Controversy:** There are debates about whether high-protein diets, including those rich in dairy, might lead to calcium loss from bones.

6. **Skin Issues:**

- **What It Is:** Some women find that consuming dairy can exacerbate skin conditions like acne.

- **Mechanism:** It's thought that the hormones and bioactive molecules in dairy can stimulate oil glands and inflammation.

7. **Weight Gain:**

- **What It Is:** *Dairy products, especially full-fat varieties, can be high in calories and fat.*

- **Potential Impact:** *Overconsumption can contribute to weight gain, which is a risk factor for several health issues including heart disease and diabetes.*

But she also discussed hormone issues, explaining how lactose can disrupt hormonal balance and wreak havoc on our gut microflora. She delved into how gut hormones impact our bodies, potentially leading to cysts, polyps, and other complications.

She didn't address the mental struggles I was facing, but that no longer seemed important.

Because it clicked. I felt a huge "bang!" in my head and thought — this might be it. Hell yeah, it must be it!

I cut out dairy immediately, ran to the lab the next day, and got tested for lactose intolerance (just to be sure).

And voila.

That was the answer. I was partly lactose tolerant.

So, my body was producing lactase, but not consistently.

Eureka!

I was over the moon — thrilled, ecstatic, and beyond words. I'd cracked the code, and everything was going to get better!

I slashed lactose from my diet as much as possible. No more morning yogurts, cheese, or cream. I also avoided ready-made cookies, cakes, sausages, desserts, and any other products packed with lactose.

After my surgery, I eagerly awaited the day when all my symptoms would finally disappear.

Symptoms

Lactose intolerance is a common digestive problem where the body is unable to digest lactose, a type of sugar found in milk and dairy products. This condition occurs due to a deficiency of lactase, an enzyme produced by the lining of your small intestine that's needed to break down lactose.

What Is Lactose Intolerance?

- **Definition:** *Lactose intolerance is the inability to digest lactose properly due to insufficient levels of lactase.*
- **Prevalence:** *It affects a significant portion of the population.*

Symptoms of Lactose Intolerance

Symptoms typically appear between 30 minutes to 2 hours after consuming dairy products and can vary in severity depending on the amount of lactose consumed and the individual's level of lactase deficiency. Common symptoms include:

- **Bloating:** *Excess gas produced by the fermentation of undigested lactose in the colon can cause a swollen, bloated feeling.*

- **Diarrhea:** *Lactose fermentation draws water into the colon, leading to watery stools.*

- **Gas:** *Fermentation of undigested lactose by bacteria in the colon produces gas, leading to flatulence.*

- **Abdominal Pain and Cramps:** *Increased gas and water in the colon can cause pain and cramping.*

- **Nausea:** *Some people may feel nauseous after consuming lactose.*

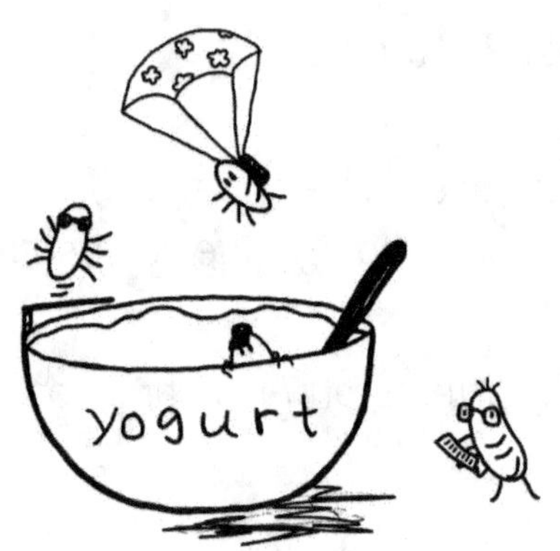

Image 14. Dairy

I have to admit, I never really had digestive issues with dairy. I mean, I didn't experience any gut discomfort — everything seemed normal to me. That's why I never thought food could be a problem. And my doctors didn't consider it either.

My symptoms were mostly mental (aside from the initial nausea years ago) and also included fatigue, breast issues, polyps and cysts. None of this was ever considered a "gut issue" — at least, I wasn't told it could be during my decade-long journey.

So, I started Googling how lactose intolerance might affect mental health.

Potential Mental Health Impacts of Lactose Intolerance

1. ***Discomfort and Stress:***
   - ***Digestive Symptoms:*** *Frequent digestive discomfort such as bloating, gas, diarrhea, and abdominal pain can cause significant physical stress.*
   - ***Mental Strain:*** *Ongoing physical discomfort can lead to increased stress and anxiety, affecting overall mental well-being.*

2. ***Dietary Restrictions:***
   - ***Social and Dietary Anxiety:*** *Avoiding dairy can limit food choices and make social eating situations challenging, potentially leading to feelings of isolation or anxiety.*
   - ***Nutritional Concerns:*** *Worry about getting enough essential nutrients like calcium and vitamin D from a restricted diet can also cause stress.*

3. ***Gut-Brain Axis:***
   - ***Gut Health and Mood:*** *The gut-brain axis is a bidirectional communication system between the gastrointestinal tract and the brain. Poor gut health, often linked to digestive disorders like lactose intolerance, can influence mental health.*

- **Microbiome Impact:** *Lactose intolerance can alter the gut microbiome, which has been shown to affect mood and mental health.*

4. **Fatigue and Low Energy:**

   - **Nutrient Absorption:** *Malabsorption of nutrients due to lactose intolerance can lead to fatigue and low energy levels, which can negatively impact mood and mental clarity.*

   - **Mental Fatigue:** *Chronic physical symptoms can also contribute to mental fatigue, making it harder to concentrate and affecting cognitive function.*

5. **Psychological Distress:**

   - **Embarrassment and Self-Esteem:** *Experiencing symptoms in social situations can cause embarrassment and lower self-esteem, particularly if symptoms are frequent or severe.*

   - **Depression and Anxiety:** *Chronic health issues, including lactose intolerance, can contribute to or exacerbate depression and anxiety.*

Inspired by this discovery, I decided to get tested for celiac disease. The test came back negative, but I learned that celiac disease can also have a significant impact on mental health. Studies show that some people suffer from depression for years, but eliminating gluten can make it disappear entirely.

I've read about one study where a woman in her 60s arrived at the hospital in terrible shape, struggling with digestive problems, depression, anxiety, and other issues for years. Doctors discovered she had celiac disease, removed gluten from her diet, and all her symptoms vanished. She became completely healthy and even managed to gain some weight.

Celiac Disease

Celiac disease is a chronic autoimmune disorder that primarily affects the small intestine. It is triggered by the ingestion of gluten, a protein found in wheat, barley, and rye. In individuals with celiac disease, consuming gluten leads to an immune response that damages the lining of the small intestine, which can interfere with nutrient absorption.

Key Aspects of Celiac Disease

1. ***Immune Response to Gluten:***
   - *When a person with celiac disease eats gluten, their immune system mistakenly attacks the villi in the small intestine. Villi are tiny, finger-like projections that help absorb nutrients from food.*

2. ***Symptoms:***
   - ***Digestive Symptoms:*** *Common symptoms include diarrhea, bloating, gas, abdominal pain, nausea, and constipation.*

- ***Other Symptoms:*** *Celiac disease can also cause symptoms beyond the digestive system, such as fatigue, weight loss, anemia, bone or joint pain, headaches, skin rashes (dermatitis herpetiformis), and neurological symptoms like numbness or tingling in the hands and feet.*

- ***Children:*** *In children, celiac disease can lead to poor growth, delayed puberty, and behavioral issues.*

Chapter 13

I cut out dairy a week before my surgery, had the procedure, and then caught COVID-19 somewhere along the way. So, after the surgery, I was sprawled on the sofa for a week, battling a high fever and other unpleasant symptoms.

I didn't notice any changes in my mental health. Everything felt the same — anxiety and fatigue persisted. A month went by, and nothing shifted. I planned to see a new gastroenterologist, recommended by my relatives, in a couple of weeks. I also wanted to give myself some time to process everything that had happened.

So, I decided to go on vacation — head to the sea, explore a new country I'd never visited before, and give myself the chance to relax, do nothing, and tune in to how my psyche was responding to the new diet.

Even though I thought I'd found the reason, I was still anxious that nothing would change. I feared I'd remain nervous and miserable forever, and that "forever" notion only made me more anxious and unhappy. On top of that, post-COVID insomnia was wrecking my evenings.

One day, while traveling — about a month and a three weeks after my discovery and surgery — I decided to try some calming hemp gummy bears. It was a pure experiment, spurred on by friends who claimed that hemp, especially in gummy form, might help with my sleep issues.

I took a handful because one or two gummies didn't seem like enough (I had tried a couple the day before). That evening, something shifted. Maybe my brain finally recognized that I wasn't poisoning myself anymore, or perhaps it was just the right moment. The next morning, I felt lighter and calmer.

I'd never felt this light and calm before, not even as a kid (I suspect I should've avoided dairy since I was 5). Suddenly, I could think clearly, listen to others, and communicate without feeling stressed. The next day, I experienced all this and wondered — is it even normal? To be calm and relaxed? To lie on the bed doing nothing and actually feel comfortable in your own skin?!

Hemp

Hemp products, particularly those containing cannabinoids like cannabidiol (CBD) and tetrahydrocannabinol (THC), can have various effects on the psyche. The impact largely depends on the specific cannabinoid content, dosage, and individual responses.

Cannabidiol (CBD)

Non-Psychoactive Effects:

- **Anxiety Reduction:** *CBD is known for its anxiolytic properties. It can help reduce anxiety and stress in some individuals by interacting with serotonin receptors in the brain.*

- **Mood Improvement:** *Some studies suggest that CBD can improve mood and alleviate symptoms of depression by influencing the endocannabinoid system and serotonin receptors.*

- **Sleep Aid:** *CBD may help improve sleep quality by reducing anxiety and promoting relaxation.*

Mechanisms of Action:

- **Serotonin Receptors:** *CBD interacts with 5-HT1A receptors, which are involved in anxiety and mood regulation.*

- **Endocannabinoid System:** *CBD modulates the endocannabinoid system, which plays a role in maintaining homeostasis, including mood and stress response.*

Tetrahydrocannabinol (THC)

Psychoactive Effects:

- **Euphoria:** *THC is the primary psychoactive component of cannabis, leading to feelings of euphoria or a "high." This effect is due to THC binding to CB1 receptors in the brain.*

- **Altered Perception:** *THC can alter perception, time sense, and sensory experiences. This can be enjoyable for some but disorienting or unsettling for others.*

- **Anxiety and Paranoia:** *In higher doses or in sensitive individuals, THC can induce anxiety, paranoia, or even panic attacks.*

Mechanisms of Action:

- **CB1 Receptors:** *THC binds to CB1 receptors in the brain, which are part of the endocannabinoid system involved in regulating mood, memory, and perception.*

That day, I wondered — what if it's just the hemp and tomorrow I wake up feeling the same old way? It was the scariest thought ever, I have to admit. Because for the first time in years (or maybe decades), I was experiencing positive thoughts and actually felt good in my body. I had never felt this way before.

I found immense joy in simply stretching my muscles, moving, standing, and walking. It was a strange, ecstatic sensation. I had always seen my body as a mere tool for survival, a means to get things done. I had never truly appreciated how wonderful it is just to be in it — to feel it. To move your fingers, stretch your legs, and release tension in your shoulders.

"I'm still high," was my next thought that day.

Plus, the hemp experience wasn't exactly a walk in the park. Before the total relaxation and falling asleep the previous evening, my anxiety shot through the roof. I have no idea how I managed to stay in my hotel room instead of running through the streets in my pajamas, screaming, "Help, my brain wants to kill me!" It was a wild ride — one of the worst experiences of my life. I promised myself I'd never use that stuff again. NEVER.

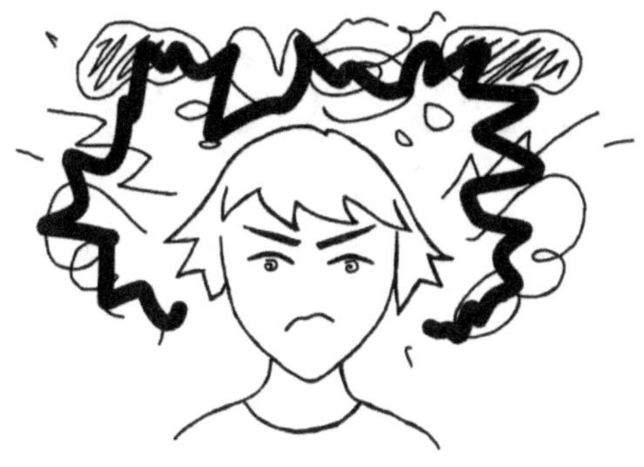

Image 15. Hemp

I was more frightened than excited. If this feeling vanished, I couldn't rely on hemp every day. The price of that feeling would be too high. My usual supercharged anxiety, magnified a thousand times, would be unbearable. That's what I was thinking.

But then I decided — I can't control all of this. All I can do is observe and wait. So, let's see what happens next.

I'd been living in constant paranoia and anxiety for so long that it was time to decide whether to push forward or to relax and breathe. Once I had that thought, my psyche calmed down a bit. After a full day of hanging out with friends, sightseeing, and walking, I finally fell asleep.

The next morning, I woke up as this new, relaxed version of myself. My anxiety was gone. I felt good, fresh, renewed, healthy — and happy?

Chapter 14

Do you know how it feels to wake up in the morning, smiling, singing a song, and being in a great mood? I do now. But I had no idea it was possible, at least for me. Theoretically, I knew there were people out there who felt this way. But honestly, I was always skeptical, thinking — maybe they're on antidepressants? Or maybe everything in their lives is perfect? Maybe they're living their dreams, with zero problems, no health issues, and enjoying only happiness, prosperity, and small wonders every day? Maybe their lives are just easier than mine?

Because when I tried to make myself calm and happy as an adult, it was all an act. I was suffering, doing my best to find joy in small things and to love life, but deep down, it was a lie. Every morning was a struggle. Every task or problem felt massive, requiring immense effort to tackle. My psyche and even my body felt the strain. Every nerve and muscle were tense, working overtime just to help me move forward. My brain was anxious and paranoid, torn apart by countless questions and problems. It was a never-ending conversation in my head.

That's why I thought it was the gummy bears' impact and why I was afraid to fall asleep and then wake up.

Because that evening in the hotel, in a foreign country, I suddenly experienced what it's like to have a happy, calm brain without suffering or that inner dialogue. It was pure joy. As if someone pushed a magic button and voila! My life wasn't perfect at all — no wonders, lots of problems, family issues, war, financial struggles — but I was totally different.

And I didn't want to lose all that.

The next morning, I was still the new me. Okay, I thought, maybe it's just the hemp and I'm still a bit high. Let's wait and see.

The next day, I stayed calm. And the next day, and the day after that.

I was still traveling, alone and amazed, feeling so much at once that it completely overwhelmed me.

It was like someone opened the door of a box I used to live in and let me see, feel, and perceive a new, bigger reality that was now my home. No boxes, no inner dialogue, just colors, smells, and feelings. I felt really good in my body, able to walk 20 kilometers and feel fine. I'd never felt that way before.

It had been 1 month and 3 weeks with no lactose in my diet.

And I couldn't believe it was even possible. I mean, I had visited numerous doctors, and not once did they mention food intolerance. I had no idea food intolerance could have such a huge impact on the human brain. And here I was — a miracle had happened in my life, and I couldn't accept it because I didn't believe it was happening to me.

To me, who had decided that suffering was my path and I had to endure it. I saw no other options but to grind and move forward somehow (with huge stones on my shoulders, like Sisyphus), but suddenly, the stones were gone.

And I realized that I had carried these stones all my life. When I was a kid, I remember coming back from school and thinking about troubles, problems, issues, and being sad all the time. I felt good around my friends, but when they weren't around, I was in a depressed state of mind. That's why I read a lot, distracting myself from sad thoughts and feelings.

I felt so sorry for that little child who endured so much, alone, with no help, support, or kind words to ease the suffering even a bit. I didn't get much kindness from my family, and now I felt sad because all that suffering could've been totally avoided if I had been tested for lactose intolerance earlier.

I was grieving that day, walking by the Baltic Sea and picking up seashells. It was a wonderful, sunny winter day; I even took off my coat because it got really warm. I thought, well, it is what it is. You were neglected then and you struggled in your 20s and 30s, but now it's time to live. I will give myself as much kindness and support as needed.

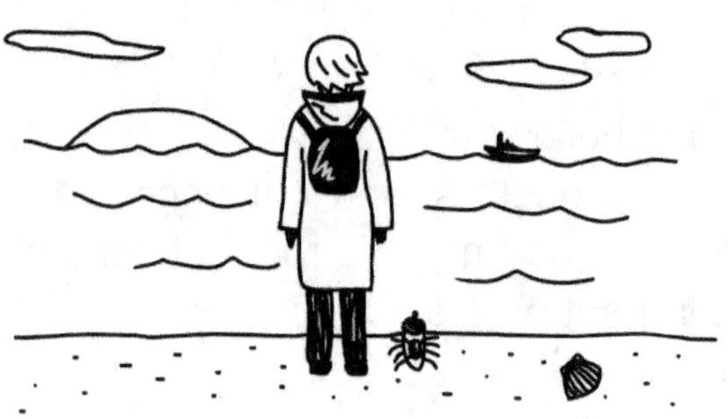

Image 16. Time to live

I was happy and upset at the same time. Because it was huge and because now, I was facing a new life, new food habits, new everything, including self-perception.

Chapter 15

I came back from my trip in March 2024, spent some time gardening and reflecting on everything that had happened to me. I was always an exceptionally compliant patient. I did everything the doctors told me to do (except taking oral contraceptives – the one thing I refused), and I visited them whenever they said. I was a good girl. And now I saw where it had brought me. I was following every instruction without questioning – and that darn yogurt nearly killed me.

Because I wasn't questioning if it was good for me. You know what – my first gynecologist was right – yogurt can really improve your microbiome and help with vaginal candidiasis.

But in my case, it was milk that ruined my health. And she had no idea (neither did I).

Yogurt and vaginal health

1. ***Beneficial Bacteria:***

   - *Yogurt contains probiotics, primarily Lactobacillus species, which are also a major component of a healthy vaginal microbiome. These beneficial bacteria help maintain an acidic environment (low pH) in the vagina, which can prevent the overgrowth of harmful bacteria and yeast.*

2. **Prevention and Treatment of Infections:**

   • *Probiotics can help in the prevention and treatment of common vaginal infections such as bacterial vaginosis (BV) and yeast infections. Lactobacillus species produce lactic acid and hydrogen peroxide, which inhibit the growth of pathogenic microorganisms.*

And I was angry, but the source of my anger wasn't that woman (a professional who had genuinely helped thousands of women), nor my other doctors. They sincerely tried to help me.

I was angry because the system was broken. We are treated like a collection of body parts. Doctors address patients as if they are just a sum of their individual parts. Family doctors often lack the knowledge to see the human body (and mind) as a whole.

It took me 10 years, countless hours of research, and one lucky coincidence (because who knew Alyona would watch that video about dairy and women's health in the first place?) to realize how amazing and complex our bodies are. And I'm not even a doctor.

But I'm truly grateful to my own patience and my brain for sticking with it despite all the anxiety and chaos. And to my body, which, despite the struggle, kept pushing forward and helping me on this journey.

I gathered all my courage and went to see the new gastroenterologist.

He was quite young and seemed genuinely intrigued when I handed him a lengthy list of symptoms that had been accumulating over the past decade (and probably my whole life).

"Depressed state, anxiety, racing thoughts, inability to concentrate, allergies..." He skimmed through the list, then looked up at me with curiosity.

"Doctor, am I sane?"

"What? Why do you ask?"

"I mean, am I normal and is my mind okay? I cut out lactose from my diet, and now all those symptoms are gone. I feel amazing. I've never felt this way before. I'm worried if my brain is functioning properly."

He chuckled.

"You're perfectly fine. In fact, we're currently seeing a patient with depression who might have the same issue as you. Lactose intolerance can cause a range of symptoms, though it varies from person to person. People can experience different symptoms in similar situations."

The relief I felt was obvious. I said:

"Oh my! That is awesome!"

The doctor smiled and replied, "You did a great job. You're on the right track. But let's take a closer look at a few other things and see how lactose might have affected you."

So, I underwent a series of tests: blood tests to check for parasites (which was a relief because at least he acknowledged that worms could be a factor), an ultrasound, and tests to investigate any inflammation in my gut and potential dysbiosis.

Dysbacteriosis, also known as dysbiosis, refers to an imbalance in the microbial communities, particularly in the gut. This imbalance can lead to a predominance of harmful bacteria over beneficial ones, affecting overall health.

Causes of Dysbacteriosis:

1. **Antibiotic Use:** Antibiotics can kill both harmful and beneficial bacteria, leading to an imbalance.

2. **Poor Diet:** Diets high in sugar, refined carbohydrates, and unhealthy fats can promote harmful bacteria growth.

3. **Stress:** Chronic stress can alter gut bacteria composition.

4. **Infections:** Gastrointestinal infections can disrupt the balance of gut bacteria.

5. **Chronic Diseases:** Conditions like diabetes, inflammatory bowel disease, and others can affect gut microbiota.

Impacts on Health:

1. **Digestive Issues:** Dysbacteriosis can cause symptoms like bloating, gas, diarrhea, constipation, and abdominal pain.

2. **Immune System Dysfunction:** The gut microbiota plays a crucial role in immune function. An imbalance can lead to a weakened immune response, making the body more susceptible to infections.

3. **Inflammation:** Dysbiosis is associated with chronic inflammation, which is a risk factor for various diseases, including cardiovascular disease, arthritis, and autoimmune disorders.

4. **Mental Health:** *The gut-brain axis links gut health to mental health. Dysbiosis has been associated with anxiety, depression, and other mood disorders.*

5. **Metabolic Disorders:** *An imbalance in gut bacteria can contribute to obesity, insulin resistance, and type 2 diabetes by affecting how the body processes food and stores fat.*

6. **Skin Conditions:** *Skin conditions like eczema, acne, and psoriasis have been linked to gut health. Dysbacteriosis can exacerbate these conditions.*

7. **Nutrient Absorption:** *Healthy gut bacteria help in the absorption of nutrients like vitamins and minerals. Dysbiosis can lead to deficiencies and malnutrition.*

Managing Dysbacteriosis:

1. **Probiotics and Prebiotics:** *Consuming foods rich in probiotics (like yogurt, kefir, and fermented foods) and prebiotics (like garlic, onions, and bananas) can help restore balance.*

2. **Healthy Diet:** *A balanced diet rich in fiber, fruits, vegetables, and whole grains supports beneficial bacteria.*

3. **Limit Antibiotics:** *Use antibiotics only when necessary and under medical guidance.*

4. ***Reduce Stress:*** *Stress management techniques like meditation, yoga, and exercise can improve gut health.*

5. ***Avoid Harmful Substances:*** *Reducing the intake of alcohol, processed foods, and artificial sweeteners can help maintain a healthy gut microbiota.*

"You did a great job."

His words echoed in my mind. They were the best words I'd ever heard.

I had done it. I had conquered the monster. I had come through this Health Journey.

I won.

I didn't have worms (I suspected I might, but I'd already had tests before). Still, I was thrilled that this doctor was actually paying attention and seemed to know his stuff.

But I did have dysbiosis. My gut was packed with harmful bacteria and lacked the good ones.

This was because I'd been eating food that didn't agree with me. I also had trouble digesting white bread, which the tests confirmed. After each surgery, I'd taken antibiotics, but my system hadn't had enough time or probiotics to recover. My liver and kidneys were "tired," and my pancreas had scars from food intolerances, as the ultrasound specialist put it.

My gallbladder wasn't in great shape either.

I also had a significant overgrowth of Proteus Mirabilis in my gut, likely spreading to other organs and systems. This bacterial invasion may explain why I dealt with kidney sand for decades.

Despite various doctors prescribing antibiotics and other medications, it wasn't until I consulted Dr. Maliarenko that the true root of my issues was uncovered.

Proteus mirabilis is a type of Gram-negative bacterium that is commonly found in the human intestinal tract, as well as in soil and water. While it is part of the normal flora in the gut, *Proteus mirabilis* can cause several types of infections, particularly when it spreads to other parts of the body.

1. *Urinary Tract Infections (UTIs)*

   - *Proteus mirabilis* is a well-known cause of UTIs, particularly in individuals with structural abnormalities of the urinary tract or those who use urinary catheters. The bacterium has the ability to produce an enzyme called urease, which breaks down urea into ammonia. This increases the pH of urine, making it more alkaline, which can lead to the formation of kidney stones.

   - *Symptoms:* UTI symptoms caused by *Proteus mirabilis* include frequent urination, burning during urination, cloudy or foul-smelling urine, and lower abdominal pain.

2. *Kidney Stones*

   - The alkaline environment created by *Proteus mirabilis* in the urinary tract can lead to the formation of struvite stones (a type of kidney stone made of magnesium ammonium phosphate). These stones can cause significant pain and may require medical intervention to remove.

- **Complications:** Large kidney stones can block the flow of urine and lead to serious complications such as kidney infections or even kidney damage.

3. **Wound Infections**

- **Proteus mirabilis** can infect wounds, especially in immunocompromised individuals or in hospital settings. It is particularly problematic in surgical wounds or bedsores.

- **Symptoms:** Wound infections may present as redness, swelling, warmth, pain, and the presence of pus or a foul-smelling discharge.

4. **Sepsis**

- In severe cases, especially when an infection spreads from the urinary tract or a wound into the bloodstream, **Proteus mirabilis** can cause sepsis. This is a life-threatening condition characterized by widespread inflammation, tissue damage, and organ failure.

- **Symptoms:** Symptoms of sepsis include high fever, rapid heart rate, rapid breathing, confusion, and low blood pressure.

5. ***Respiratory Infections***

- *Although less common,* **Proteus mirabilis** *can also cause respiratory tract infections, particularly in hospitalized patients or those with underlying lung conditions.*

6. ***Complications in Women's Health***

- **Proteus mirabilis** *has been implicated in infections of the female reproductive system, particularly in association with urinary tract infections. Chronic infections or inflammation caused by* **Proteus mirabilis** *could potentially contribute to conditions such as pelvic inflammatory disease (PID), which may lead to complications like chronic pelvic pain or infertility if left untreated.*

Antibiotic Resistance

- *One of the significant concerns with* **Proteus mirabilis** *is its increasing resistance to multiple antibiotics. It can produce extended-spectrum beta-lactamases (ESBLs) that break down a wide range of antibiotics, making infections difficult to treat.*

Prevention and Treatment

- **Prevention:** *Good hygiene practices, especially in hospital settings, and proper management of urinary catheters can reduce the risk of infection.*

> **Treatment:** *Treatment typically involves the use of antibiotics, but the choice of antibiotic may depend on the susceptibility of the specific strain of* **Proteus mirabilis** *causing the infection.*

I also discovered that Proteus Mirabilis can contribute to mood swings and significantly impact mental health. And honestly, I was shocked. Not only because no one had ever mentioned this connection to me before, but also because, looking back at my life, I realized that I had been living under the alien influence of wrong food and bacteria for so long. This invisible invader was disrupting my life, draining the joy and happiness from it, and turning me into an anxious, robotic version of myself—like a human without the essence of being alive inside.

This realization was devastating. I felt an overwhelming sense of grief and pain.

> • **Proteus mirabilis** *can potentially cause mental symptoms and affect mood, although it's not as commonly discussed as other gut-related issues.* **Proteus mirabilis** *is a type of bacteria that can contribute to urinary tract infections (UTIs), which can lead to systemic inflammation. This inflammation can sometimes affect the brain, leading to changes in mood, cognition, and overall mental health.*

- *Infections and chronic inflammation in the body are known to impact the gut-brain axis, the communication pathway between the gut and the brain. When this axis is disrupted, it can lead to mental symptoms such as anxiety, depression, brain fog, and mood swings. Additionally, the stress of dealing with chronic health issues like recurrent infections can also have a psychological impact, further affecting mood and mental well-being.*

- *So, while **Proteus mirabilis** itself isn't directly linked to mental symptoms, the inflammation and systemic effects caused by an overgrowth of this bacteria can indirectly contribute to mood changes and mental health issues.*

I got a 3-month treatment plan and went home. Despite taking antibiotics for a while, I'd never felt this good before. Within a month, I felt even better. I was out in the garden, battling sweltering summer temperatures of +35°C, and still managing just fine. I'm pretty sure I'd have been toast under those conditions two years ago.

My physical health was on the up and up, and my mind was calm and focused.

Chapter 16

All the puzzles

But that one jar of homemade yogurt kept me thinking.

When I was a kid, visiting the village during holidays often brought on strange symptoms (besides the frequent food poisoning). My fingers would swell up, I'd feel off, and I had odd reactions to solar eclipses and weather changes. Not to mention the breast issue.

My grandmas cooked with plenty of butter and used a lot of dairy. Their meals were packed with lactose: bread, pies, pancakes, loads of white flour with milk or cream, and cottage cheese pies. It was lactose overload every single day.

What if all my symptoms were signs that the food I was eating was just wrong for me?

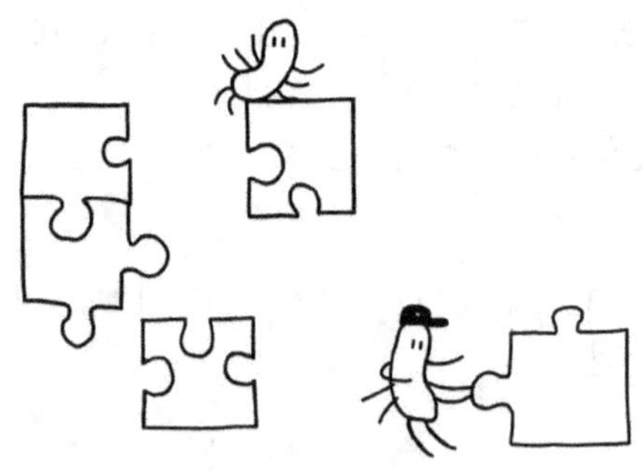

Image 18. Puzzles

Suddenly, the bigger picture started to make sense.

Whenever I ate more dairy, I felt worse. It wasn't just the dairy itself; it was in everything — from cheese to ready-made products. My body was trying to tell me something was off, especially when I had vaginal candidiasis, but I didn't listen.

I think my gut's hormonal balance was already out of whack after my divorce, and things just got worse with the yogurt and additional dairy I was consuming.

It wasn't anyone's fault; sometimes, we just don't know what we don't know.

Food intolerances can have a wide range of consequences on both the human body and psyche. Unlike food allergies, which involve an immune response, food intolerances are typically related to the digestive system's inability to process certain foods properly. Here are some of the key consequences:

Physical Consequences

1. ***Gastrointestinal Issues:***
   - *Bloating and Gas: Incomplete digestion can lead to fermentation in the intestines, causing gas and bloating.*
   - *Diarrhea or Constipation: Food intolerances can disrupt normal bowel movements, leading to diarrhea or constipation.*
   - *Abdominal Pain and Cramping: Ingesting intolerant foods can cause significant discomfort and cramping.*

2. **Nutrient Deficiencies:**

   - *Malabsorption: Chronic inflammation and digestive issues can impair the absorption of essential nutrients, leading to deficiencies.*

   - *Weight Loss or Gain: Nutrient malabsorption can cause unintended weight loss, while some people may gain weight if they eat excessive amounts of safe foods to compensate.*

3. **Inflammation:**

   - *Chronic Inflammation: Persistent ingestion of foods that the body cannot tolerate can lead to chronic inflammation, which is linked to various health conditions, including arthritis and cardiovascular diseases.*

4. **Skin Problems:**

   - *Rashes and Eczema: Food intolerances can manifest as skin issues, including rashes, eczema, and acne.*

5. **Headaches and Migraines:**

   - *Frequent Headaches: Certain food intolerances, like those to tyramine or caffeine, can trigger headaches and migraines.*

Psychological Consequences

1. **Mood Disorders:**

   - *Anxiety and Depression: Chronic physical discomfort and nutrient deficiencies can contribute to the development of mood disorders such as anxiety and depression.*

- *Irritability and Mood Swings: Ongoing digestive issues and discomfort can lead to increased irritability and mood swings.*

2. **Cognitive Issues:**

- *Brain Fog: Difficulty concentrating, memory problems, and overall cognitive impairment can result from chronic inflammation and nutrient deficiencies.*

3. **Stress and Social Impact:**

- *Social Isolation: Managing food intolerances can be stressful, leading to social withdrawal due to the fear of eating out or attending social events.*

- *Stress and Anxiety: The constant need to monitor and avoid certain foods can create significant stress and anxiety.*

I think my brain was trying to send me a warning. My body had other symptoms, signaling that something was off, but since they weren't gut-related, I didn't have a clue about what was going on. And honestly, no one really knows why this happens. Each of us reacts differently to things that are bad for us. Some people might never figure it out — like my mother, who took the test after me and discovered she was also completely lactose intolerant — but never felt any issues. Others, like me, are hypersensitive. But this heightened sensitivity didn't make it any easier to pinpoint the right diagnosis.

My psyche was sensing something, but I had no idea what it was trying to tell me. Different symptoms are our body and mind's way of responding to irritants, substances, viruses, bacteria, and so on. It's like a universal language that our body-mind team speaks, and we need to learn how to understand it. That's exactly what I'm working on now — figuring out how to communicate with my own body and mind.

Although I'm not a doctor, I've gained a lot of knowledge about the human body and mind. I can now interpret some blood tests and know when to stay alert and where to seek help. It's not good or bad — it's just part of taking responsibility for your own health.

I'm also really glad I decided against taking oral contraceptives. I have no idea what kind of impact they might have had on my health, but given the state I was in, I can only imagine how it could've made things worse. My body was already struggling and not functioning properly, so those hormones wouldn't have been a solution — they'd have just masked the symptoms.

Chapter 17

The most eye-opening discovery from my Health Journey is how many diseases — and even deficiencies like a lack of vitamin D — can present with psychological symptoms that often get mistaken for depression. Our bodies and brains are constantly trying to communicate their issues. We might experience overwhelming anxiety that can be resolved with something as simple as an antihistamine pill (like my spring allergies, for instance). It could be a hormone imbalance. Or it might be due to a worm or bacteria.

So, the key takeaway is this: if you're feeling anxious and depressed, get your blood tested, check your hormones, food intolerances, bacteria, and allergies. For instance, I've learned that my spring allergies trigger anxiety, and it disappears as soon as I take an antihistamine pill — that's how I know what's happening now. I didn't realize this before, but now my brain signals me, saying, "I'm anxious, irritated, and not feeling great; please check that little rash on your feet." And I listen.

Many diseases can manifest psychological symptoms such as depression and anxiety. These symptoms can arise due to the direct impact of the disease on the brain and nervous system, the stress of dealing with chronic illness, or side effects of treatments. Here are some diseases and conditions that can present with psychological symptoms:

Chronic Physical Illnesses

1. ***Cardiovascular Diseases:***

   - *Heart Disease and Stroke: Patients often experience depression and anxiety due to the impact on lifestyle and fear of future cardiac events.*

2. ***Diabetes:***

   - *Type 1 and Type 2 Diabetes: The daily management of diabetes, as well as blood sugar fluctuations, can contribute to mood swings, depression, and anxiety.*

3. ***Chronic Pain Conditions:***

   - *Fibromyalgia, Arthritis, and Migraines: Chronic pain is a significant risk factor for depression and anxiety.*

4. ***Gastrointestinal Disorders:***

   - *Irritable Bowel Syndrome (IBS) and Inflammatory Bowel Disease (IBD): These conditions are often linked to depression and anxiety due to ongoing discomfort and the impact on daily activities.*

Neurological and Neurodegenerative Diseases

1. ***Multiple Sclerosis (MS):***

   - *MS can directly affect the brain, leading to depression, anxiety, and cognitive changes.*

2. ***Parkinson's Disease:***

- *Depression and anxiety are common due to both the neurochemical changes in the brain and the physical limitations caused by the disease.*

3. ***Alzheimer's Disease and Other Dementias:***

- *These conditions can cause mood disturbances, depression, and anxiety as cognitive decline progresses.*

4. ***Epilepsy:***

- *Seizures and the side effects of anticonvulsant medications can lead to mood disorders.*

Autoimmune and Endocrine Disorders

1. ***Thyroid Disorders:***

- *Hypothyroidism and Hyperthyroidism: Both conditions can cause significant mood changes, including depression and anxiety.*

2. ***Systemic Lupus Erythematosus (SLE):***

- *The chronic nature and systemic impact of lupus can lead to psychological symptoms.*

3. ***Rheumatoid Arthritis:***

- *Chronic inflammation and pain, as well as the impact on mobility and daily function, can result in depression and anxiety.*

Infectious Diseases

1. ***HIV/AIDS:***
   - *The psychological impact of diagnosis, stigma, and the chronic management of the disease can lead to depression and anxiety.*
2. **Chronic Hepatitis C:**
   - *The long-term nature of the disease and its treatment can cause mood disturbances.*
3. **Post-Influenza or Post-Viral Syndromes:**
   - *Conditions like post-viral fatigue syndrome can lead to ongoing psychological symptoms.*

Brain tumors

- *Tumors in the brain can directly impact mood and cognitive function.*

Metabolic and Nutritional Disorders

1. ***Vitamin Deficiencies:***
   - *Deficiencies in vitamins such as B12, D, and folate can lead to symptoms of depression and anxiety.*
2. **Electrolyte Imbalances:**
   - *Conditions that affect electrolyte balance, such as chronic kidney disease, can result in mood changes.*

Chronic Fatigue Syndrome (CFS) and Myalgic Encephalomyelitis (ME)

1. *CFS/ME:*

   - *These conditions are characterized by extreme fatigue and can be accompanied by depression and anxiety due to their impact on daily life.*

Now I also know, that food intolerances may cause depressive states too. And of course, parasites.

The Impact of Parasites on Human Mental Health

These organisms impact on human health, including mental well-being. These organisms can cause a variety of physical and psychological symptoms, often leading to significant distress.

1. **Direct Impact on the Brain:** *Some parasites can directly invade the central nervous system. For example, Toxoplasma gondii, a common parasite, can infect the brain and alter neurotransmitter levels, potentially leading to mood disorders such as depression and anxiety.*

2. **Immune Response and Inflammation:** *The body's immune response to parasitic infection can lead to chronic inflammation. This inflammation has been linked to various mental health issues, including depression, anxiety, and cognitive impairments. The ongoing immune response can alter brain function and chemistry, contributing to these symptoms.*

3. **Nutritional Deficiencies:** *Parasites can cause malabsorption of essential nutrients by damaging the gut lining. Nutritional deficiencies, particularly in vitamins and minerals crucial for brain health, can lead to cognitive decline, mood disorders, and decreased mental function.*

4. **Gut-Brain Axis Disruption:** *The gut-brain axis is a bidirectional communication system between the gastrointestinal tract and the brain. Parasites disrupting the gut microbiome can affect this communication pathway, leading to changes in mood, behavior, and cognitive function. The imbalance in gut bacteria can produce neuroactive substances that influence mental health.*

5. **Stress and Psychological Burden:** *Living with a parasitic infection can be psychologically taxing. The chronic nature of some infections, coupled with the physical symptoms, can lead to increased stress, anxiety, and depression. The stigma and social isolation associated with certain parasitic diseases can further exacerbate mental health issues.*

6. **Sleep Disturbances:** *Parasitic infections can cause significant sleep disturbances due to itching, pain, or general discomfort. Poor sleep quality and insomnia are closely linked to mental health problems, including depression and anxiety. The lack of restorative sleep can impair cognitive function and emotional regulation.*

Understanding the link between parasitic infections and mental health is crucial for comprehensive medical care. Addressing parasitic infections not only improves physical health but can also lead to significant improvements in mental well-being.

They don't teach this stuff in school. Thanks to Wikipedia and the Internet, I've learned a lot about the human body and mind, and how they're connected.

By the end of 2023, I'd done a bunch of blood tests to check for various diseases. I took this on myself because doctors were convinced I was fine. But I'm stubborn. When I get that nagging feeling that something's off, I dig in because I know the truth is hiding in that tiny gut instinct.

I shared some of what I found with Alyona, and as you can see, it worked. She played a huge role in saving my sanity — and maybe even my life.

And now, as I write this book, I'm amazed that I didn't see the obvious — the jar of homemade yogurt sitting on my table every morning. How did I miss it?

That was my blind spot. Food intolerances aren't a hot topic where I'm from. You won't find tons of info about them, and you definitely don't get Instagram ads screaming, "Dairy makes you anxious!" Plus, coconut yogurt isn't exactly easy to find in every supermarket. But that's another story.

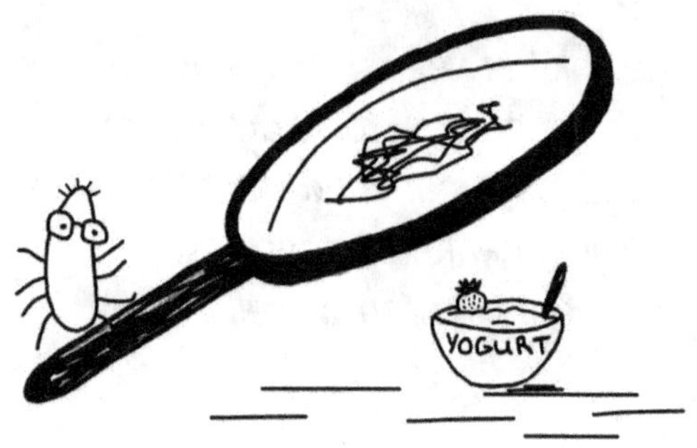

Image 19. Blind spot

My generation, I guess, was the most neglected and over-medicated one ever. As a kid, antibiotics were practically a staple. Got the flu? Here you go. Spring allergies? Oh, that must be a nasal infection — antibiotics for you. Over and over again, for years.

Meanwhile, I was never tested for food allergies or spring allergies. I shudder to think about the state of my microbiome and gut after all that. Ugh, it's terrifying. But here I am — survived it all! I navigated this crazy journey, conquered the monster, and wrapped up my Health Journey.

Actually, not quite over yet — my dysbacteriosis is still hanging around. But, thank goodness, I'm not anxious anymore. I'm working on getting better.

Chapter 18

My doctor also explained that the gut-brain axis is a crucial system linking the gut and the brain, influencing both mental and physical health. In my case, the anxiety I experienced was significantly related to the state of my gut microbiome. The imbalance of bacteria in my gut, often referred to as dysbiosis, was exacerbated by consuming foods that were harmful to me.

Bad bacteria in the gut thrive on certain types of food, and their proliferation can disrupt normal gut function. This disruption can lead to systemic inflammation and influence neurotransmitter production, which in turn affects brain function and mood. Essentially, the bad bacteria were contributing to my anxiety by affecting this vital communication network between my gut and brain.

Gut-Brain Axis

1. *The gut-brain axis refers to the complex bi-directional communication network linking the gastrointestinal (GI) tract and the central nervous system (CNS). This pathway involves multiple mechanisms through which the gut and brain influence each other, impacting both physiological and psychological processes.*

2. **Neuroanatomical Pathways:** The gut-brain axis involves direct and indirect connections between the gut and the brain. The vagus nerve is a primary conduit for this communication, transmitting signals between the gut and the brainstem. Additionally, the enteric nervous system (ENS), often termed the "second brain," consists of a network of neurons embedded in the gut wall that can operate independently of the central nervous system.

3. **Microbiome Influence:** The gut microbiome, composed of trillions of microorganisms residing in the GI tract, plays a crucial role in the gut-brain axis. Microbial metabolites, such as short-chain fatty acids, can influence brain function and behavior by modulating neuroinflammation and neurotransmitter production. Dysbiosis, an imbalance in the gut microbiome, has been associated with various neuropsychiatric disorders, including anxiety and depression.

4. **Immune System Interactions:** The gut-associated lymphoid tissue (GALT) is an integral component of the gut-brain axis, interacting with the immune system to influence brain function. The gut microbiome can affect systemic inflammation, which in turn can impact brain health and contribute to neuroinflammatory conditions.

5. ***Endocrine Pathways:*** *Hormonal signals from the gut, including stress-related hormones like cortisol and gastrointestinal hormones such as ghrelin and leptin, can affect brain function and mood. These hormonal interactions are part of the broader endocrine system influencing the gut-brain axis.*

6. ***Psychological Implications:*** *The gut-brain axis plays a role in regulating emotional and cognitive functions. Research has shown that disturbances in this axis may contribute to mental health disorders, such as irritable bowel syndrome (IBS), anxiety, and depression.*

So I ditched the wheat flour and processed foods. I went bread-free for three months and carefully chose sausages (I'm a sausage fan — if you offer me cake or sausage, sausage wins every time). I made sure they were lactose-free and included mostly meat, with no soy or other ingredients. I explored seven different types of flours, whipping up banana-coconut-oatmeal pancakes and even baked a coconut cake (pricey compared to dairy, but totally worth it).

I mostly stuck to simple, homemade meals — think fruits, veggies, meat, fish, oatmeal, rice, potatoes, nuts (goodbye cookies and snacks), and greens. I cut back on caffeine and had zero alcohol during this time (actually I haven't been drinking it for years but still). Water was my go-to, with the occasional juice. I even discovered lactose-free candies and energy bars, though I only indulged now and then since I'm not a big sugar fan. I brewed buckwheat tea, enjoyed chicory (which I love), and mixed in coconut or almond milk. I also treated myself to coconut yogurts from the supermarket now and then.

I took probiotics and some pricey pills for my liver and gall-bladder. My breast pain completely disappeared (I could hardly believe it, but it was true). The soreness in my fingers was gone. I could finally focus on conversations and dive back into my hobbies. My mind was clear, and my mood was fantastic.

The ultrasound specialist, who was also a gastroenterologist, was astonished. She asked, "What treatment did your doctor prescribe? Your internal organs look completely different from three months ago. They're healthy."

My doctor did his magic.

My body did its magic.

We did magic together.

You're welcome to join my community, where you can explore health insights, share your stories, and ask questions. I'll be posting regular updates on my health journey, discoveries, and thoughts on how transforming your diet can transform your life. Let's take care of our health and explore wellness together!

www.irynakhmara.space

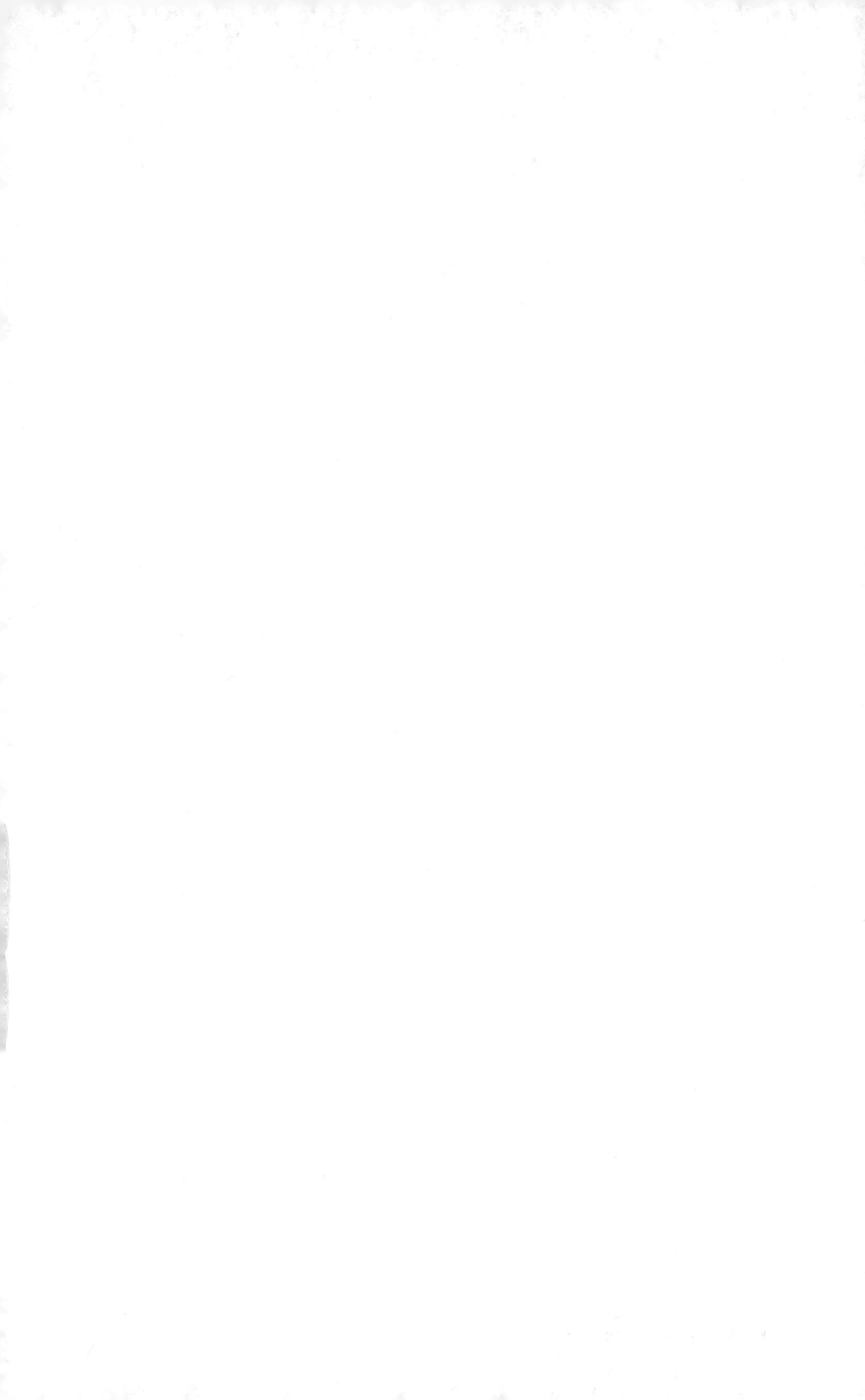